Guidelines on Neonatal Seizures

WHO Department of Mental Health and Substance Abuse

WHO Department of Maternal, Newborn, Child and Adolescent Health

OASI Department of Mental Retardation Unit of Neurology and Clinical Neurophysiopathology

IRCCS Associazione Oasi Maria SS. WHO Collaborating Centre

International League Against Epilepsy ILAE Established 1909

EPILEPSY out of the shadows A Global Campaign Against Epilepsy

World Health Organization

WHO Library Cataloguing-in-Publication Data: 2011

Guidelines on neonatal seizures.

1.Seizures - diagnosis. 2.Seizures - prevention and control.
3.Seizures - drug therapy. 4.Infant, Newborn, Diseases.
5.Guidelines. I.World Health Organization.
ISBN 978 92 4 154830 4 (NLM classification: WS 421)

Editing: Rosa Di Giorgio

Graphics: Leonardo Arangio

Printed in Italy - Villaggio Cristo Redentore srl, Troina EN - Tel. +39 0935 657813

TABLE OF CONTENTS

Abbreviations

AED	antiepileptic drug
CI	confidence interval
CNS	central nervous system
CRD	Centre for Reviews and Dissemination
CT	computed tomography
DARE	Database of Abstracts of Reviews of Effects
EEG	electroencephalography
GDG	Guideline Development Group
GRADE	Grading of Recommendations Assessment, Development, and Evaluation
HIE	hypoxic-ischaemic encephalopathy
IBE	International Bureau for Epilepsy
ILAE	International League Against Epilepsy
IMCI	Integrated Management of Childhood Illness
IMPAC	Integrated Management of Pregnancy and Childbirth
IRCCS	Institute for Research on Mental Retardation and Brain Aging
ISRCTN	International Standard Randomized Controlled Trial Number Register
MD	mean difference
mRCT	meta-register of randomized controlled trials
MRI	magnetic resonance imaging
MRS	magnetic resonance spectroscopy
NGO	non-governmental organization
NLM	National Library of Medicine
NPV	negative predictive value
NS	neonatal seizures
OR	odds ratio
PPV	positive predictive value
PT	preterm
RCT	randomized controlled trial
RR	relative risk
US	ultrasound
WHO	World Health Organization
WMD	weighted mean difference

Executive Summary

Neonatal seizures represent one of the most frequent neurological events in newborn infants, often reflecting a variety of different pre-, peri-, or postnatal disorders of the central nervous system (CNS). They are also a common manifestation of metabolic abnormality in newborn period and often represent the first sign of neurological dysfunction in neonates. They may be symptomatic or cryptogenic, herald subsequent epilepsy, can be associated with potential morbidity and mortality, and may be used as a factor in considering long-term prognosis. Despite the enormous clinical significance of these events, many aspects of their management are not well supported with evidence-based recommendations.

In particular, rather few studies address issues related to the use of antiepileptic drugs (AEDs), such as indications for acute therapy, selection of first-line and second-line agents, pharmacokinetics of commonly used AEDs, and duration of treatment after the seizures are controlled on AEDs for neonatal seizures (NS).

The Global Campaign Against Epilepsy, a World Health Organization (WHO) partnership with the International League Against Epilepsy (ILAE) and the International Bureau of Epilepsy (IBE), in collaboration with the Institute for Research on Mental Retardation and Brain Aging (IRCCS) named Associazione Oasi Maria SS., a WHO Collaborating Centre for Training and Research in Neuroscience (WHO/CC), initiated a project to develop evidence-based guidelines for the management of neonatal seizures. These guidelines are intended to be of use for neonatologists, paediatric neurologists, paediatricians, general practitioners, nurse practitioners, nurses and other health professionals who may be in contact with infants experiencing seizures within the first 28 days of life (age up to 44 weeks post-conception). The guidelines are framed so as to be applied by health care providers practicing in a wide range of health care facilities, from those with limited resources to tertiary care centres.

The Guideline Development Group identified 11 research questions to be of highest priority. Two of these questions were background questions on prevalence of neonatal seizures and predictors of prognosis of neonatal seizures. The remaining 9 questions focused on priority issues related to management of neonatal seizures. The Grading of Recommendations Assessment, Development, and Evaluation (GRADE) approach was used for grading the quality of evidence after adaptation to the relevant working area. The quality of the evidence for an outcome was graded as follows: high, moderate, low or very low. After grading the available studies for each outcome, recommendations were formulated on the basis of the summary and quality of evidence, balance between benefits and harms, values and preferences of policy makers, health care providers and parents, feasibility and resource use; in addition, costs were analyzed to see whether they could be qualitatively justifiable by the benefits. The recommendations were graded into two types: *strong* and *weak*. In some cases, the recommendations were *context-specific* which is indicated in the document as appropriate.

Table 1 lists the key recommendations of the guidelines:

TABLE 1- KEY RECOMMENDATIONS OF NEONATAL SEIZURES GUIDELINES

No.	RECOMMENDATIONS	Strength	Quality of evidence
1.	Clinically apparent seizures in the neonate should be treated if they last more than 3 minutes or are brief serial seizures.	*Strong*	*Not graded*
	In specialized care facilities where electroencephalography is available, all electrical seizures, even in the absence of clinically apparent seizures, should also be treated.	*Strong, context-specific*	*Not graded*
2.	In all neonates with seizures, hypoglycaemia should be ruled out and treated if present before antiepileptic drug treatment is considered.	*Strong*	*Not graded*
	If facilities for measuring glucose are not available, consider empirical treatment with glucose.	*Weak, context-specific*	
	If there are clinical signs suggestive of associated sepsis or meningitis, central nervous system infection should be rule out by doing a lumbar puncture, and treated if present with appropriate antibiotics.	*Strong*	
	If facilities for lumbar puncture are not available, consider empirical treatment with antibiotics for neonates with clinical signs of sepsis or meningitis.	*Weak, context-specific*	
	In all neonates with seizures, serum calcium should be measured (if facilities are available) and treated if hypocalcaemia is present.	*Strong, context-specific*	
	In the absence of hypoglycaemia, meningitis, hypocalcaemia or another obvious underlying etiology such as hypoxic-ischaemic encephalopathy, intracranial haemorrhage or infarction, pyridoxine treatment may be considered before antiepileptic drug treatment in a specialized centre where this treatment is available.	*Weak, context-specific*	
3.	Phenobarbital should be used as the first-line agent for treatment of neonatal seizures; phenobarbital should be made readily available in all settings.	*Strong*	*Very low*
4.	In neonates who continue to have seizures despite administering the maximal tolerated dose of phenobarbital, either a benzodiazepine, phenytoin or lidocaine may be used as the second-line agent for control of seizures (use of phenytoin or lidocaine requires cardiac monitoring facilities).	*Weak*	*Very low*
5.	In neonates with normal neurological examination and/or normal electroencephalography, consider stopping antiepileptic drugs if neonate has been seizure-free for >72 hours; the drug(s) should be reinstituted in case of recurrence of seizures.	*Weak*	*Very low*
6.	In neonates in whom seizure control is achieved with a single antiepileptic drug, the drug can be discontinued abruptly without any tapering of the doses.	*Weak*	*Not graded*
	In neonates requiring more than one antiepileptic drug for seizure control, the drugs may be stopped one by one, with phenobarbital being the last drug to be withdrawn.	*Weak*	
7.	In the absence of clinical seizures, neonates with hypoxic-ischaemic encephalopathy need not to be given prophylactic treatment with phenobarbital.	*Strong*	*Moderate*
8.	Where available, all clinical seizures in the neonatal period should be confirmed by electroencephalography.	*Strong, context-specific*	*Not graded*
	Electroencephalography should not be performed for the sole purpose of determining the etiology in neonates with clinical seizures.	*Strong*	
9.	Radiological investigations (ultrasound, computed tomography and magnetic resonance imaging) of the cranium/head should not be performed to determine the presence or absence of clinical seizures or to evaluate the efficacy of treatment with antiepileptic drugs in neonates.	*Strong*	*Not graded*
	Radiological investigations may be done as a part of the comprehensive evaluation of the etiology of neonatal seizures or to determine prognosis in neonates with seizures.	*Weak, context-specific*	

INTRODUCTION

Seizures are a common occurrence in both term and preterm (PT) neonates. Despite their frequency and clinical significance, currently there are no clearly defined evidence-based guidelines to address major questions about their management. While diagnosis and management of seizures are often considered within the context of tertiary care health centres, seizures are a common manifestation in newborns presenting to the full range of health-care facilities. Therefore, there is a need for evidence-based guidelines which can be applied to different health-care facilities with varying resources and adapted by health-care providers of all levels of expertise.

Neonatal seizures, one of the most frequent neurological events in newborn infants, reflect a variety of pre-, peri- or postnatal disorders of the central nervous system (CNS). These may range from benign, self-limited illnesses to severe, prolonged or life-threatening disorders. They are also a common manifestation of metabolic abnormality or infection. Due to the increased availability of diagnostic tools, such as electroencephalography (EEG), video-EEG monitoring, and early neuroimaging to supplement clinical observation, the diagnosis of neonatal seizures may be established more accurately. It is also possible that incidence figures may have changed in recent times. Furthermore, higher incidence and prevalence rates of epilepsy have been found in developing countries, so it is conceivable that incidence and prevalence rates of neonatal seizures could rather differ between developed and developing countries (Brown et al., 1972; Leveno et al., 1989; Okan et al., 1995; Garcias Da Silva et al., 2004; Sankar et al., 2007).

Some aspects of treatment of neonatal seizures have changed little over the last 50 years. In newborns with seizures, it is indicated to initiate a early diagnostic work up to determine the cause, depending upon the facilities available. Even though most neonates who present with seizures are treated with antiepileptic drugs (AEDs), only very few studies address the issues related to use of AEDs such as the first-line and second-line drugs, their pharmacokinetics, the duration of treatment, and the methods of discontinuing treatment after achieving adequate control of seizures. In particular, there is a lack of randomized controlled trials to validate a treatment algorithm of neonatal seizures. The AEDs used tend to be older generation drugs associated with the most side effects (Co et al., 2007). Moreover, clinical control of neonatal seizures using the two commonly used AEDs - phenobarbital and phenytoin - is achieved in only 50 to 80% of cases, with even less effect in the control of most neonatal electrical seizures (Painter et al., 1999; Boylan et al., 2002; Rennie et al., 2003; Boylan et al., 2004). Management of neonatal seizures becomes even more difficult in resource-poor settings because of the limited number of facilities available for diagnosis, treatment and monitoring.

Clinical and experimental data suggest a longer duration of seizures as being associated with greater difficulty in controlling them. Furthermore, seizures can have immediate and long-term adverse consequences on the immature and developing brain (Shany et al., 2007). Irrespective of immediate attempts to suppress the neonatal seizures with AEDs, the risk for subsequent neuro-developmental deficits and early death is substantial. Newborn infants with seizures are at risk for death, whereas survivors are at risk for neurological impairment, developmental delay, later epilepsy and cognitive impairment (Ronen et al., 2007). Hence, it is important to conduct systematic review of the evidence to determine the optimal diagnosis and treatment regimens for the management of neonatal seizures.

Scope of Guidelines and Target Audience

These guidelines have been produced in response to a request for guidance to managing of neonatal seizures, with the hope of highlighting as well as resolving some of the controversies in this field, and to standardize practice.

All health workers involved in the care of the newborn infant are commonly confronted with the clinical problem of seizures in neonates. Despite the frequency of these events, that can be acute, symptomatic or herald subsequent epilepsy, no clear answers are currently available to major questions about their management nor are there evidence-based guidelines for the management of neonatal seizures.

However, the clinical concerns go beyond those raised by physician-specialists. Health-care providers with varying degrees of training have to face the issues of newborns with seizures, irrespective of the level of resources available at the facility they are working at. The lack of guidelines for care in these settings is also an important health-care problem to be addressed.

Accordingly, the Global Campaign Against Epilepsy, a World Health Organization (WHO) partnership with the International League Against Epilepsy (ILAE) and the International Bureau of Epilepsy (IBE), in collaboration with the Institute for Research on Mental Retardation and Brain Aging (IRCCS) named Associazione Oasi Maria SS., a WHO Collaborating Centre for Training and Research in Neuroscience (WHO/CC), conducted systematic review of the literature to assist in developing evidence-based guidelines for the management of neonatal seizures. The WHO Departments involved in the development of these guidelines included the Department of Mental Health and Substance Abuse and the Department of Maternal, Newborn, Child and Adolescent Health. The WHO/CC Associazione Oasi Maria SS. (IRCCS), based in Troina (EN), Italy, provided financial support for the development of guidelines and the organization of relevant meetings.

These guidelines are intended to be of use for neonatologists, paediatric neurologists, paediatricians, general practitioners, nurse practitioners, nurses and all the other health professionals that may be responsible for addressing problems of newborns with seizures occurring within the first 28 days of life (up to 44 weeks post-conception). The document has been written so that it can be applied to care-givers practicing at a wide range of health care facilities: from those with limited resources to those functioning as tertiary care centres.

Methodology

The Guideline Development Group (GDG) was convened to advise on the content and process, interpretation of evidence and to formulate and finalize the recommendations. It consisted of experts with multidisciplinary expertise and with an adequate regional and gender representation. Multidisciplinary expertise that was sought included guideline development methodology, neonatology, paediatrics, paediatric neurology, primary care, public health and epidemiology. A list of GDG members is provided in **Annex 1**.

Declaration of conflict of interest

A conflict of interest declaration as per WHO rules was filled by all contributors. Helen Cross (United Kingdom) reported receiving travel support for herself to attend meetings (£5000) and honoraria for educational activities (£5000 for herself plus the research unit) from Eisai, UCB and Janssen Cilag (in total combined) and being on the advisory board of Eisai and UCB (£1000). Angelina Kakooza (Uganda) received international scholarship award in 2005 for a 6-week fellowship in Boston from the American Epilepsy Society as well as support from said Society to attend Society meetings in 2005 and 2007. Hans Hartmann (Germany) reported owning company shares in Pfizer for US$10000 and Novartis for US$15000. The other members of the GDG reported no conflict of interest. The declared conflicts of interest were reviewed by the technical units and discussed with the Director of the responsible unit. During the meeting, all members provided a verbal summary of their written declarations of interest. None of the declared interest by the GDG members were considered significant as to affect the proceedings of the GDG and for any further action to be taken.

Formulating questions and choosing outcomes

At the first GDG meeting held in Troina, Sicily, Italy, on November 16-17, 2007, key questions requiring an answer were drafted. The scoping questions focused on controversial areas that needed to be covered or topics requiring changes in policy or practice. In addition to the scoping questions, outcomes were identified for evidence review and making decisions and recommendations. These were rated as critical, important or not important by the GDG members. Each of the questions deserved separate systematic reviews, taking into consideration the critical and important outcomes. The performed systematic reviews were peer-reviewed by the GDG and also by external peer-reviewers.

Priority questions

The following questions were identified to be of the highest priority:

Background questions

- What is the prevalence of various causes of neonatal seizures in different geographical regions of the world?
- Which clinical factors and diagnostic tests best predict the prognosis of neonatal seizures?

Questions directly related to management of neonatal seizures

1. Which newborn seizures require acute antiepileptic drug treatment?
2. What is the clinical efficacy of empirical treatment of newborns with seizures (prior to laboratory tests) for hypoglycaemia, hypocalcaemia, and bacterial infection/meningitis?
3. Which is the preferred first-line antiepileptic drug for a newborn with seizures requiring treatment with antiepileptic drugs?

4. Which is the preferred second-line antiepileptic drug treatment for a newborn with seizures not responding to maximal tolerated dose of phenobarbital?

5. If a newborn has seizures and is controlled on current antiepileptic drug treatment, when should the medication be discontinued?

6. If a newborn has seizures and is controlled on current antiepileptic drug treatment, how should the medication be discontinued?

7. What is the effect of prophylactic treatment of at-risk neonates with hypoxic-ischaemic encephalopathy on mortality, recurrence of seizures and/or long-term neurological outcomes?

8. What is the value of electroencephalography in the management of a newborn with seizures?

9. What is the value of imaging of the cranium/head in diagnosis, evaluation of etiology, treatment, and prognosis of the newborn with seizures?

Evidence retrieval and synthesis

Selection of studies

We searched all published trials utilizing random or quasi-random patient allocation as well as observational studies for useful information related to the priority questions. Recent review articles were also searched to ensure inclusion of specific references relevant to the question. For the question on epidemiology of neonatal seizures (NS), we also referred to national chapters of International League Against Epilepsy (ILAE) – the international professional epilepsy non-governmental organization (NGO) – to get information on country-based databases and any prevalence studies on NS that may not have been published in indexed journals.

Type of participants

Full-term neonates with clinical and/or electrographic seizures, commencing within the first 28 days of life and preterm neonates presenting with clinical and/or electroencephalograhic seizures commencing before a corrected age of 28 days (44 weeks postconception).

Search strategy, data abstraction and synthesis of the evidence

Literature search was performed using all key words consecutively. The explored databases are enclosed in the **Appendix.** Studies were stratified according to type of intervention or exposure, study design, birth weight and gestational age where possible. Effects were expressed as relative risks (RR) or odds ratios (OR) for categorical data and as mean differences (MD) or weighted mean differences (WMD) for continuous data wherever possible. When available, results adjusted for potential confounders – particularly for observational studies – were preferred to unadjusted results. When results adjusted for potential confounders were not available, unadjusted results were used. All the studies reporting on a critical outcome are summarized in the table of individual studies (**Annex 2**).

Grading the quality of evidence

We considered pooled effects for developing recommendations, wherever feasible. When results of three or more randomized controlled trials (RCTs) were available for an outcome, and the overall quality of evidence using the Grading of Recommendations Assessment, Development, and Evaluation (GRADE) approach was at least "low", observational studies were not considered. However, when there were 2 or less RCTs for an outcome or the quality of evidence was "very low", we pooled the effects from RCTs with those from available cohort and case-control studies. When pooled effects were available from published systematic reviews and no new studies were identified, we used the published pooled effects. When considering new studies, we updated the pooled effects using "metan" command in Stata 11.0. The same was done when no published pooled effects were identified. For pooling, we used the author reported adjusted effect sizes and confidence intervals as far as possible. We used random effects models for meta-analysis either when important inconsistency in effects was found or random effects model was not unduly affected by small studies. When pooling of results was not possible, we used the range of effect sizes observed in the individual studies in developing recommendations.

All relevant reviews were summarized and the evidence was synthesized using the GRADE methodology where possible (Atkins et al., 2004). In case it was not possible to GRADE the evidence, a study-by-study table was developed to summarize and assess the quality of the evidence. **Annex 2** provides the evidence synthesis.

A few pragmatic instructions and adaptations to guide the application of GRADE were developed to increase consistency by ensuring that the same background logic was employed in assessing the evidence for each scoping question. These instructions were used to rate the five aspects considered in the quality assessment: (1) limitations (risk for bias); (2) inconsistency; (3) indirectness; (4) imprecision; (5) reporting bias. The quality of the set of studies included – reporting results for an outcome – was graded as: high, moderate, low or very low. The interpretation of the above grades in these guidelines is the following:

High: One can be sure that the intervention is beneficial, has no effect or is harmful. Results, including the magnitude of the pooled effect, are unlikely to change with new studies.

Moderate: One can be reasonably sure that the intervention is beneficial, has no effect or is harmful. However, the magnitude of the pooled effect may change with new studies.

Low: Although it is likely, one cannot be sure the intervention is beneficial, has no effect or is harmful. The magnitude of the pooled effect is uncertain and is likely to change with new studies.

Very low: One cannot be certain about the effects of the intervention.

One of the difficulties in using GRADE is that the evidence base for an outcome may include studies with varying methodological quality and sample size. We therefore included the weight of the studies in the estimation of the pooled effect to make judgments about the quality of the set of included studies. The criteria used to grade the quality of evidence are shown in Table 2. We used a cut-off of 50% of total weight of evidence for rating the study design, limitations in methods, and directness. For consistency, we used a cut-off of 75% of total weight.

TABLE 2 - GRADE CRITERIA FOR ASSESSING THE QUALITY OF EVIDENCE

Design Based on design of studies with ≥50% of weight of evidence	**Limitations in Methods** Based on methods of studies with ≥50% of weight of evidence			**Analysis intention to treat; cluster adjusted if applicable** *(adjusted for confounding)*	**Precision**	**Consistency**	**Directness**	**Overall Quality of Evidence**
	Allocation concealment *(the two comparable groups and low risk of reverse causality)*	**Blinding or other approaches to reduce measurement bias**	**Loss to follow-up**		Based on 95% CI of the pooled effect size	Based on the direction of effect size of ≥2 studies with ≥75% of weight of evidence	Based on directness of studies with ≥50% of weight of evidence	Based on the score total in columns on the left
If RCT, then = 0 If quasi-RCT, then = -0.5 *(If observational, then = -1.0)*	If allocation concealment adequate, then = 0 If allocation concealment inadequate / unknown, then = -0.5 Not applicable if quasi-randomized *(If observational studies with important risk of selection bias or reverse causality, then = -0.5)*	If blinding to intervention, then = 0 If “objective” outcome, then = 0 If outcome not “objective” but observers blinded, then = 0; if not, then = -0.5 If difference in measurement procedures for the two comparison groups, then = -0.5	If cohort followed up, and <20% lost, then = 0; if not, then = -0.5 If representative cross sectional surveys, then = 0; if not, then = -0.5	If intent to treat analysis, then = 0; if not, then = -0.5 If cluster RCT and analysis cluster-adjusted, then = 0; if not, then = -0.5 *(If observational studies adjusted for confounding then = 0, if not, then= -0.5)*	If CI does not include “null”, and both CI limits mean meaningful benefit or unacceptable harm, then= 0 If CI does not include “null”, but CI wider than above, then= -0.5 If CI includes “null”, and both CI limits exclude meaningful benefit or unacceptable harm, then= 0 If CI includes “null”, but CI wider than the above, then= -1.0	If ≥3 studies and pooled effect indicates meaningful benefit or unacceptable harm, and individual studies in the same direction as pooled effect, then= 0, if not, then= -1.0 If ≥3 studies and pooled effect indicates no effect, and individual studies also indicate no effect, then = 0, if not, then= -1.0 If only two studies with effect sizes in same direction, then = -0.5, if effect sizes in different directions, then= -1.0 If single study, then= -1.0	If population as well as intervention in studies same as those of interest, then = 0 If one of the two different from that of interest , then = -0.5 If both different from those of interest, then = -1.0	If final score = 0 or -0.5, then **HIGH** If final score = -1 or -1.5, then **MODERATE** If final score = -2 or -2.5, then **LOW** If final score ≤-3, then **VERY LOW**

Formulation of recommendations

The second GDG meeting was organized on March 6-8, 2009 to draft and finalize the recommendations. A two-step process was followed to draft the recommendations. First, the evidence was summarized and quality of evidence assessed for all the questions. The GDG then considered the summary and quality of evidence, balance between benefits and harms, values and preferences of policy-makers, health care providers and parents, feasibility and resource use; in addition, costs were analyzed to see whether they could be qualitatively justifiable by the benefits to formulate the recommendation for all the questions, irrespective of the GRADE being used for assessing the quality of evidence. On the basis of considerations on the balance between desirable and undesirable effects, quality of evidence, values, preferences and feasibility issues, the GDG additionally provided a judgment on the strength of each recommendation, to be categorized as *strong* or *weak*. We anticipated that, in some circumstances, recommendations may apply only if specific conditions are met. Indeed, they were context-specific recommendations, as indicated for the recommendations where relevant.

The strength of a recommendation reflects the degree of confidence to the extent that the desirable effects of adherence to a recommendation outweigh the undesirable effects. Desirable effects can include beneficial health outcomes, less burden and savings. Undesirable effects can include harms, more burden and higher costs. Burdens are the demands of adhering to a recommendation that patients or caregivers (e.g. families) may dislike, such as having to undergo more frequent tests or opting for a treatment that may require a longer time for recovery.

Although the degree of confidence is a continuum, the GRADE system defines two categories: ***strong*** and ***weak***.

- A *strong* recommendation is one for which the panel is confident that the desirable effects of adherence to a recommendation outweigh the undesirable effects. This can be either in favour of or against an intervention.
- A *weak* recommendation is one for which the panel concludes that the desirable effects of adherence to a recommendation probably outweigh the undesirable effects, but the panel is not confident about these trade-offs. Reasons for not being confident can include:
    - › absence of high quality evidence
    - › presence of imprecise estimates of benefits or harms
    - › uncertainty or variation in how different individuals value the outcomes
    - › small benefits
    - › the benefits may not be worth the costs (including the costs of implementing the recommendation).

Despite the lack of a precise threshold between a strong and a weak recommendation, the presence of important concerns about one or more of the above reasons makes a weak recommendation more likely. In addition, some of the recommendations were ***context-specific***, i.e. some recommendations, be strong or weak, might not be applicable in all settings.

Implications of a strong recommendation are as follows:

- For patients: most people in this situation would want the recommended course of action and only a small proportion would not.
- For clinicians: most patients should receive the recommended course of action. Adherence to this recommendation is a reasonable measure for good quality care.
- For policy makers: the recommendation can be adopted as a policy in most situations. Quality initiatives could use this recommendation to measure variations in quality.

Implications of a weak recommendation are as follows:

- For patients: the majority of people in this situation would want the recommended course of action, but many would not.

- For clinicians: be prepared to help patients to make a decision that is consistent with their own values.
- For policy makers: there is a need for substantial debate and involvement of stakeholders.

Consensus, external review and updating

The scoping questions and outcomes as well as the evidence reviews were circulated for peer-review to experts from different regions of the world. An audit was kept for all the comments received from the external reviewers; comments were discussed and agreed upon by the GDG members.

During the meetings, the designated member of the GDG presented the systematic review of the evidence, balance between benefits and harms, values and preferences, resource use and feasibility issues. All the above issues were discussed by the GDG for each of the scoping questions. Agreement was reached by consensus. The "review by date" was discussed by GDG members and it was decided that Department of Mental Health and Substance Abuse will review the guidelines for any update required 5 years after its publication.

Presentation, dissemination, and implementation plan

A print and electronic version of the guidelines will be published for wider dissemination and easy access for the target audiences. In addition, the guidelines would be disseminated by partners involved in its development through their networks. Articles based on the guidelines would also be submitted to journals for its wider dissemination to scientific audience.

The guidelines will be field-tested in different health settings and by different cadres of health care providers before its implementation. Following the field test and any necessary revisions, guidelines will be considered for inclusion in the standard WHO training materials, including the Integrated Management of Childhood Illness (IMCI), the Integrated Management of Pregnancy and Childbirth (IMPAC), and Pocketbook for Hospital Care for Children.

Summary of questions and recommendations

Background question

What is the prevalence of various causes of neonatal seizures in different geographical regions of the world?

Table 3 - Prevalence of neonatal seizures

Study population	Date of publication of studies	Prevalence of different etiologies in infants with neonatal seizures (%)			
		Hypoxic-ischaemic encephalopathy	Hypoglycaemia	Hypocalcaemia	Central Nervous System Infections
Term neonates	<1990	48% (13 to 83) [3 studies]	5.5% (5 to 6.5) [3 studies]	9% (2.6 to 20) [3 studies]	10.3% (9.5 to 12) [2 studies]
	≥1990	38% [1 study]	-	-	7.5% [1 study]
Preterm neonates	<1990	40% [1 study]	3% [1 study]	2.3% (1.5 to 3) [2 studies]	5.5% (5 to 6) [2 studies]
	≥1990	-	-	-	-
Both term and preterm OR unknown gestation	<1990	42.5% (12.5 to 77) [16 studies]	6% (1 to 13) [7 studies]	6% (0.5 to 43) [10 studies]	10% (0.7 to 24) [14 studies]
	≥1990	40% (12 to 80) [10 studies]	7.5% (4 to 13) [2 studies]	5% (5 to 5) [2 studies]	8.5% (2 to 16) [8 studies]

*Median (range); see **Annex 2** for details of individual studies*

Note: Data stratified by date of publication (before and after 1990) because of the availability of better monitoring and diagnostic modalities that could help in easy identification of studies in the latter period

Salient findings

- Given the differences in characteristics of the underlying populations, study designs, study sites, and classification and definitions used, it is difficult to provide a single estimate of the prevalence of different disease conditions in neonates with seizures.
- Among neonates with seizures, the reported ranges of median prevalence are the following: hypoxic-ischaemic encephalopathy (HIE): 38-48%; hypoglycaemia: 3-7.5%; hypocalcaemia: 2.3-9%; central nervous system (CNS) infections: 5.5-10.3% (see Table 3).
- The prevalence of these four common etiologies do not appear to be different between term and preterm neonates. Also, we did not find any rate differences between the studies published before and after 1990.
- Studies have reported higher frequency of neonatal seizures (NS) in males than in females as well as in Black rather than in White infants or infants from other ethnicities and in preterm babies (Bergman et al., 1983; Saliba et al., 1999; Saliba et al., 2001).
- Most of the studies were conducted in developed country settings, with only very few studies conducted in developing countries.

Background question

Which clinical factors and diagnostic tests best predict the prognosis of neonatal seizures?

Summary of evidence – Salient findings

- Studies included in the review mainly provided a moderate level of evidence because of the limitations in study populations, study design, and insufficient duration of the clinical follow-up and sparse data. Also, lack of electroencephalography (EEG) confirmation in some studies might influence the study results because of inclusion of neonates with electro-clinical and clinical seizures of possible non-epileptic events. All studies, except for one, were conducted in developed countries, in settings well equipped to accurately diagnose and monitor seizures and therapy, and to assess the outcomes. Therefore, all the findings might not be applicable in settings with limited resources (see **Annex 2** for details of individual studies).

- In general, prognosis and outcomes of NS are determined by neurological examination during infancy and later in life, long-term neurodevelopment, and presence of the post-neonatal epilepsy. The most reliable early predictors of later neurological outcomes are the underlying etiology of the seizures and specific EEG background patterns.

- Multiple rather than single factors seem to be most accurate in predicting outcome. Nearly all variables relate to the degree of brain injury at the time of seizure occurrence which, in turn, relates to etiology.

- The interictal EEG from one or serial recordings, the ictal EEG and findings on neuroimaging are selected as most powerful methods for NS prognosis. Background EEG activity is significantly and independently related to the neurodevelopment outcome.

- An abnormal neurological examination appears to be related to an adverse outcome as well. Since this parameter is independent from any diagnostic equipment, it should be a part of the follow-up plan for infants with neonatal seizures in any settings.

- As preterm neonates appear to have a higher risk for long-term adverse outcome than term infants with NS, they have to be followed more closely for abnormal neurological development.

- Different, standardized instruments are available for assessment of neurodevelopment in infants; they could be adapted to the specific population. The age-appropriateness and the quality of expertise are crucial for their quality and reliability.

- The effects of antiepileptic drugs (AEDs) on the immature and developing brain are not clear. There is no convincing data that short-term or long-term therapies adversely alter cognitive function. No study addressing this issue was found.

- Concerning the limitations of nonrandomized, cohort or observational studies, a prospective, multicentre, randomized placebo-controlled trial with long term clinical follow-up of neurological and cognitive outcomes is recommended. Instruments of the assessment should be adapted to the low-resource settings.

QUESTION 1

Which newborn seizures require acute antiepileptic drug treatment?

Summary of evidence – Values and benefits

- In newborns with seizures, work-up should be initiated quickly to determine the cause, depending upon the facilities available. We did not identify any randomized controlled trials or well conducted observational studies examining the effects of AED treatment compared with no treatment in infants with NS.
- There is some evidence from observational studies that serial, ongoing seizures are detrimental to the developing brain; there is also some evidence that electrical seizures may be associated with worse outcome if not controlled.
- Though a significant clinical benefit has not been demonstrated in the past, the possible benefits of treatment with AEDs outweigh possible harms with no evidence of clinically relevant adverse effects of adequate and short term AED treatment.

Recommendation(s)

- Clinically apparent seizures in the neonate should be treated if they last more than 3 minutes or are brief serial seizures (strong recommendation).
- In specialized care facilities where electroencephalography is available, all electrical seizures, even in the absence of clinically apparent seizures, should also be treated (strong, context-specific recommendation).

QUESTION 2

What is the clinical efficacy of empirical treatment of newborns with seizures (prior to laboratory tests) for hypoglycaemia, hypocalcaemia, and bacterial infection/meningitis?

Summary of evidence – Values and benefits

- There is no evidence from trials to support or reject empirical treatment (prior to laboratory tests) for hypoglycaemia, hypocalcaemia and bacterial or viral infections.

- The prevalence of hypoglycaemia in neonates with seizures is 3-7.5% (Table 3). Hypoglycaemia can be deleterious and is associated with sequelae including epilepsy (Caraballo et al., 2004). A risk/benefit analysis of empirical treatment of hypoglycaemia is not available. The possible harm with treatment is the worsening of hyperglycaemia in some neonates with HIE. Since blood glucose can easily be measured at low cost, this should be performed before treatment.

- The prevalence of hypocalcaemia in neonates with seizures varies between different studies with a range of 2.3-9% (Table 3). The studies reporting high incidences were published in the 1970s (Keen & Lee, 1973, and Langevin, 1974). With better nutritional management, the incidence of hypocalcaemia may since have declined. However, the data available are not sufficient to prove this assumption. Measurement of blood calcium is possible in hospital settings without time delay, although less easily available than measurement of blood sugar. When given intravenously, calcium may cause significant harm, i.e. asystole or skin necrosis. The benefit *vs.* harm ratio for empirical treatment of hypocalcaemia before laboratory tests cannot be assessed.

- Data on different etiologies of neonatal seizures are highly inconsistent (Table 3). There is not sufficient evidence to describe regional differences. The only available study from an African country found a very high incidence of bacterial infections in neonates with seizures admitted to a hospital in Kenya (Idro et al., 2008). This study may be biased because only infants referred to hospital were included. The authors did not state whether the neonates showed other clinical signs of infection and gave no information about laboratory tests performed. Since oral treatment of neonatal sepsis or pyogenic meningitis is not considered as a standard therapy, empirical treatment would imply intravenous therapy.

- Congenital herpes simplex virus infection is a rare cause of NS. A population-based case-control study found an increased odds ratio of 2.9 for a history of vaginal delivery/maternal herpes simplex infection in infants presenting with seizures within the first 72 hours of life (Hall et al., 2006). The authors did not state whether the neonates showed other clinical signs of infection. Since oral treatment of congenital herpes simplex virus infection is not considered as a standard therapy, empirical treatment would imply intravenous therapy. A benefit *vs.* harm ratio of such treatment cannot be assessed due to paucity of data.

- Pyridoxine dependent epilepsy is a rare disease with an incidence of about 1:396 000 (Been et al., 2005) compared to the overall incidence of neonatal seizures between 1:71 and 1:1000. Other treatable neonatal epileptic encephalopathies with metabolic causes, such as pyridoxal-phosphate dependent epilepsy, probably are even less frequent. The diagnosis of pyridoxine dependent epilepsy can be established clinically by a positive response to treatment with pyridoxine. Failure to diagnose this condition may have deleterious effects on affected neonates, but delay in treatment of other underlying etiologies may also cause harm. A benefit *vs.* harm ratio of empirical treatment with pyridoxine cannot be calculated.

Recommendation(s)

- In all neonates with seizures, hypoglycaemia should be ruled out and treated if present, before anti-epileptic drug treatment is considered (strong recommendation).

- If facilities for measuring glucose are not available, consider empirical treatment with glucose (weak, context-specific recommendation).

- If there are clinical signs suggestive of associated sepsis or meningitis, central nervous system infection should be ruled out by doing a lumbar puncture, and treated if present with appropriate antibiotics (strong recommendation).

- If facilities for lumbar puncture are not available, consider empirical treatment with antibiotics for neonates with clinical signs of sepsis or meningitis (weak, context-specific recommendation).

- In all neonates with seizures, serum calcium should be measured (if facilities are available) and treated if hypocalcaemia is present (strong, context-specific recommendation).

- In the absence of hypoglycaemia, meningitis, hypocalcaemia or another obvious underlying etiology, such as hypoxic-ischaemic encephalopathy, intracranial haemorrhage or infarction, pyridoxine treatment may be considered before antiepileptic drug treatment, in a specialized centre where this treatment is available (weak, context-specific recommendation).

Question 3

Which is the preferred first-line antiepileptic drug for a newborn with seizures requiring treatment with antiepileptic drugs?

Summary of evidence – Values and benefits

- Commonly used first-line AEDs for treatment of NS are phenobarbital and phenytoin.
- There is very low quality evidence from a single randomized controlled trial (RCT) that the two drugs are equally effective (Table 4); it should, however, be noted that only about 55% of newborns respond to either of the two medications.
- Phenobarbital is easier to administer with a one daily dose being sufficient following attainment of therapeutic levels. Phenytoin has more severe adverse effects than phenobarbital including cardiac side effects and extravasation (although these have been mitigated by the introduction of fosphenytoin). The therapeutic range of phenytoin is very narrow and blood levels need to be measured to a greater degree than phenobarbital.
- Phenobarbital is also cheaper and more easily available than phenytoin.

Recommendation(s)

- Phenobarbital should be used as the first-line agent for treatment of neonatal seizures; phenobarbital should be made readily available in all settings (strong recommendation).

Table 4 - First-line antiepileptic drugs for neonatal seizures: GRADE profile summary

OUTCOME	No. of studies	Design	Limitations in methods	Precision	Consistency	Generalizability/ Directness	Overall Quality of Evidence	Pooled effect size (95% CI) *or range of effect sizes if pooling not possible at all*
Seizure control	1	RCT (0)	Limitations in allocation of subjects and blinding (-1.0)	Effect not significant, with wide CI (-1.0)	Single study (-1.0)	From developed country setting (-0.5)	**VERY LOW** (Total score = -3.5)	RR 0.97 (0.54, 1.72)

*See **Annex 2** for detailed GRADE profiles and tables of individual studies*

Summary of evidence – Values and benefits

- We identified only one observational study that compared midazolam with phenytoin as the second-line AED. The quality of evidence was graded as very low. There was a significant benefit in seizure control with midazolam as the second-line AED; there was, however, no benefit or harm in the long-term neurodevelopmental outcomes (Table 5).

- Two studies have examined the effects of lidocaine and benzodiazepines on seizure control. The quality of evidence was very low. There was no difference between the two (Pooled RR: 1.78, 95% CI: 0.90 to 3.52). No significant effect was observed on the long-term neurodevelopment either (Table 5).

- Compared to benzodiazepines, lidocaine has a narrow therapeutic range and also requires cardiac monitoring while being administered. Moreover, it may not be readily available in all settings. On the other hand, benzodiazepines have a higher risk in causing respiratory depression. Phenytoin also requires cardiac monitoring during administration.

Recommendation(s)

- In neonates who continue to have seizures despite the administering of the maximal tolerated dose of phenobarbital, either a benzodiazepine or phenytoin or lidocaine may be used as the second-line agent for control of seizures, the use of phenytoin or lidocaine requiring cardiac monitoring facilities (weak recommendation).

Question 4

Which is the preferred second-line antiepileptic drug treatment for a newborn with seizures not responding to maximal tolerated dose of phenobarbital?

TABLE 5 - SECOND-LINE ANTIEPILEPTIC DRUGS FOR NEONATAL SEIZURES: GRADE PROFILE SUMMARY

OUTCOME	No. of studies	Design	Limitations in methods	Precision	Consistency	Generalizability / Directness	Overall Quality of Evidence	Pooled effect size (95% CI) or *range of effect sizes if pooling not possible at all*
Benzodiazepines vs. Phenytoin								
Seizure control	1	Observational (-1.0)	Limitations in allocation of subjects, blinding, and analysis (-1.5)	Effect significant; lower limit of CI meaningful (0)	Single study (-1.0)	From developed country setting (-0.5)	**VERY LOW** (Total score = -4.0)	RR 2.13 (1.48, 3.08)
Normal neuro-development (until 1 year)	1	Observational (-1.0)	Limitations in allocation of subjects, blinding, and analysis (-1.5)	Effect not significant, with wide CI (-1.0)	Single study (-1.0)	From developed country setting (-0.5)	**VERY LOW** (Total score = -5.0)	RR 1.15 (0.62, 2.14)
Lidocaine vs. Benzodiazepines								
Seizure control	2 (1 RCT and 1 observational)	Majority of evidence from observational (-1.0)	Limitations in allocation of subjects, blinding, and analysis (-1.5)	Pooled effect not significant, with wide CI (-1.0)	Both studies in the same direction (0)	Both from developed country settings (-0.5)	**VERY LOW** (Total score = -4.0)	RR 1.78 (0.90, 3.52)
Normal neuro-development	2 (1 RCT and 1 observational)	Majority of evidence from observational (-1.0)	Limitations in allocation of subjects, blinding, and analysis (-1.5)	Pooled effect not significant, with wide CI (-1.0)	Only 2 studies, both in opposite direction (-1.0)	Both from developed country settings (-0.5)	**VERY LOW** (Total score = -5.0)	RR 1.20 (0.36, 3.96)

*See **Annex 2** for detailed GRADE profiles and tables of individual studies*

Summary of evidence – Values and benefits

- Evidence from observational studies suggests that a large proportion of neonates in whom the seizure control is achieved and who have normal findings on neurological examination, EEG, neuroimaging or combination thereof are at a low risk (< 10%) for recurrence of seizures (Table 6). Normal neurological examination includes normal sensorium and ability to breastfeed, and absence of abnormal findings in formal neurological examination; normal EEG means absence of spikes and normal background activity.

- There is very low quality evidence for significant benefits in seizure recurrence and for no benefits or harms in other outcomes like epilepsy, cerebral palsy or developmental delay following stoppage of AEDs compared with continuing therapy in neonates (Table 6).

- Given the saving on costs for both parents and health care systems, policy-makers and health providers are likely to give a high value to stopping AEDs in the neonatal period.

- No information is available regarding the time interval between achieving seizure control and discontinuing AEDs; the seizure-free interval suggested here (72 hours) is largely based on expert opinion.

Recommendation(s)

- In neonates with normal neurological examination and/or normal electroencephalography, consider stopping antiepileptic drugs if seizure-free for >72 hours; the drug(s) should be reinstituted in case of recurrence of seizures (weak recommendation).

QUESTION 5

If a newborn has seizures and is controlled on current antiepileptic drug treatment, when should the medication be discontinued?

Table 6 - Discontinuation of antiepileptic drugs in neonatal seizures: GRADE profile summary

OUTCOME	No. of studies	Design	Limitations in methods	Precision	Consistency	Generalizability/ Directness	Overall Quality of Evidence	Pooled effect size (95% CI) or *range of effect sizes if pooling not possible at all*
Seizure recurrence	3	All observational (-1.0)	Limitations in selection of subjects and analysis (-1.0)	Pooled effect significant but upper limit of CI in the 'null' range (-0.5)	All studies in the same direction (0)	All from developed country setting (-0.5)	**VERY LOW** (Total score = -3.0)	RR 0.66 (0.47, 0.93)
Epilepsy in infancy	1	Observational (-1.0)	Limitations in selection of subjects and analysis (-1.0)	Effect not significant, with wide CI (-1.0)	Single study (-1.0)	From developed country setting (-0.5)	**VERY LOW** (Total score = -4.5)	RR 0.54 (0.25, 1.19)
Cerebral palsy	1	Observational (-1.0)	Limitations in selection of subjects and analysis (-1.0)	Effect not significant, with wide CI (-1.0)	Single study (-1.0)	From developed country setting (-0.5)	**VERY LOW** (Total score = -4.5)	RR 0.63 (0.31, 1.27)
Developmental delay	1	Observational (-1.0)	Limitations in selection of subjects and analysis (-1.0)	Effect not significant, with wide CI (-1.0)	Single study (-1.0)	From developed country setting (-0.5)	**VERY LOW** (Total score = -4.5)	RR 0.91 (0.64, 1.29)

*See **Annex 2** for detailed GRADE profiles and tables of individual studies*

Question 6

If a newborn has seizures and is controlled on current antiepileptic drug treatment, how should the medication be discontinued?

Summary of evidence – Values and benefits

- There is no available data to suggest that gradual withdrawal of AEDs has effects on short term outcome such as breakthrough seizures and mortality as well as on long term outcomes, e.g. epilepsy or neurodevelopmental impairment.
- There is no data regarding the sequence of withdrawal of AEDs in the case of neonate who has had seizures and is controlled on multiple AEDs.
- The current treatment practices with regard to the mode of discontinuing AED treatment appears to vary widely between different settings and countries.
- Due to paucity of data, the following recommendations were formulated based on expert opinion.

Recommendation(s)

- In neonates in whom seizure control is achieved with a single antiepileptic drug, the drug can be discontinued abruptly without any tapering of the doses (weak recommendation).
- In neonates requiring more than one antiepileptic drugs for seizure control, the drugs may be stopped one by one, with phenobarbital being the last drug to be withdrawn (weak recommendation).

Question 7

What is the effect of prophylactic treatment of at-risk neonates with hypoxic-ischaemic encephalopathy on mortality, recurrence of seizures and/or long-term neurological outcomes?

Summary of evidence – Values and benefits

- We identified two studies – one RCT and one observational – that evaluated the effect of prophylactic therapy on mortality in infants with HIE. The quality of evidence was graded as very low. There was no significant effect on mortality (pooled RR: 1.80, 95% CI: 0.78 to 4.19). A 1.80 RR with wide confidence intervals means that we cannot entirely rule out a significant harm in mortality with prophylactic phenobarbital treatment (Table 7).

- We found two RCTs studies examining the effect of the prophylactic therapy on abnormal neurological outcome. One study reported the outcome at discharge, while the other reported the incidence at 3 years of age. The quality of evidence was graded as moderate. The pooled effect was 56% (95% CI: 24% to 79%) reduction in the risk of abnormal neurological outcome. The fact that the significant pooled effect essentially comes from a single study, however, decreases the confidence in this outcome (Table 7).

- We identified 4 studies - three RCTs and one observational - that looked at the effect of the above therapy on the incidence of seizures during the initial hospital stay. These studies used different doses of phenobarbital (10 to 40 mg/kg). The quality of evidence was graded as very low. There was no difference in the risk of subsequent seizures (pooled RR: 0.84, 95% CI: 0.34 to 2.09; Table 7).

- There is a debate about adverse effects of AEDs on the developing brain but no evidence from clinical studies. No prophylactic therapy would avoid additional medication and associated costs. Given these considerations and low-to-very low quality evidence for not significant benefits in important outcomes, policy-makers and health providers are unlikely to give a high value to prophylactic treatment with phenobarbital.

Recommendation(s)

- In the absence of clinical seizures, neonates with hypoxic-ischaemic encephalopathy do not need to be given prophylactic treatment with phenobarbital (strong recommendation).

TABLE 7 - PROPHYLACTIC TREATMENT OF AT-RISK NEONATES WITH HYPOXIC-ISCHAEMIC ENCEPHALOPATHY: GRADE PROFILE SUMMARY

OUTCOME	No. of studies	Design	Limitations in methods	Precision	Consistency	Generalizability / Directness	Overall Quality of Evidence	Pooled effect size (95% CI) *or range of effect sizes if pooling not possible at all*
Mortality (during initial hospital stay)	2 (1 RCT and 1 observational)	Majority of evidence from observational study (-1.0)	Limitations in selection of subjects and analysis (-1.0)	Pooled effect not significant, with wide CI (-1.0)	Both studies in the same direction (0)	Both studies from developing country settings (0)	**VERY LOW** (Total score = -3.0)	RR 1.80 (0.78, 4.19)
Abnormal neurological outcome (at discharge in 1 study, at 3 years in the other)	2	RCTs (0)	Limitations in follow-up and analysis (-1.0)	Pooled effect significant and lower limit of CI meaningful (0)	Only 2 studies, effect size of both in same direction (-0.5)	Majority of evidence from the study in developing country setting (0)	**MODERATE** (Total score = -1.5)	RR 0.44 (0.24, 0.79)
Incidence of seizures (in the initial hospital stay)	4 (3 RCTs and 1 observational)	Majority of evidence from RCTs (0)	Limitations in allocation of subjects, follow-up, and analysis (-1.5)	Pooled effect not significant, with wide CI (-1.0)	Effect size of studies with <75% of total weight in the same direction as pooled effect (-1.0)	Majority of evidence from studies in developing country settings (0)	**VERY LOW** (Total score = -3.5)	RR 0.84 (0.34, 2.09) Random-effects model

*See **Annex 2** for detailed GRADE profiles and tables of individual studies*

QUESTION 8

What is the value of electroencephalography in the management of a newborn with seizures?

Summary of evidence – Values and benefits

Prospective studies. *Prospective cohort studies (Ronen et al., 2007; Tekgul et al., 2006; Ortibus et al., 1996; Pisani et al., 2008b; Plouin et al., 1981; Dreyfus-Brisac et al., 1981; Bye et al., 1997) have reported an association between NS and abnormal neurological outcome, morbidity, and mortality; similarly, Mizrahi & Kellaway (1987) and Rowe et al. (1985) noted that EEG characteristics can help determine etiology and outcomes. One study (McBride et al., 2000) observed an association between the amount of electrographic seizure activity and subsequent mortality and morbidity in infants at risk for seizures and in infants with perinatal asphyxia. Normal EEG in the neonatal period has been reported to have a sensitivity of 96% and a specificity of 81% in predicting the absence of seizures in the first two years of life (Laroia et al., 1998); another study (Kerr et al., 1990) found that EEG can help predict persistence of seizures. While some studies (Scarpa et al., 1983; Kumar et al., 2007; Bye & Flanagan, 1995) noted that the use of EEG could help with anticonvulsant management, others (Connell et al., 1989) showed mixed results to this regard.*

Retrospective studies. *Several studies (Khan et al., 2008; Pisani et al., 2008a; Carrascosa et al., 1996) have reported an association between abnormal EEG findings and neurological outcome, including developmental delay, epilepsy and death. While one study (Van Rooij et al., 2007) noted that the duration – but not background pattern – was associated with neurodevelopmental outcome, other studies (Staudt, 1990; Domenech-Martinez et al., 2003) reported a good correlation between abnormal background activity and prognosis. Serial EEGs (Tharp et al., 1981) as well as EEG on the first day of life (Pezzani et al., 1986) have also been reported to help determine long-term prognosis.*

- EEG is the most accurate method for confirming that a clinical event is of epileptic origin, which is consistent with values and preferences of accurate diagnosis. However, the standard method of diagnosis is the clinical recognition of neonatal seizures.

- The risk of performing an EEG on a neonate is minimal, predominantly related to transient discomfort and scalp irritation.

- While performing EEG, certain factors need to be considered such as minimally acceptable standard for the equipment and facilities, minimal training requirements for EEG technicians and interpretation of EEG by a trained person.

- The cost for performing an EEG (purchase and instrumentation maintenance, purchase of supplies, personnel) may overwhelm health care facilities with limited resources; net benefits are context-specific. In general, the net benefits are worth the costs.

- The application of EEG to determine specific etiological factors is rather limited. Although there are some EEG patterns that may be specific for certain neonatal brain disorders, these conditions are very few, represent a small proportion of risk factors and are no longer the critical diagnostic test for these disorders. Although the relative harm of performing an EEG is negligible, there appears to be no benefit in performing the EEG for this purpose alone when other more definitive testing is available (such as neuroimaging or infectious disease diagnostics).

- Although the sequence of response to AEDs has been described by observational studies, the effect has not been quantified. Studies titrating AED therapy to elimination of electrographic seizures have not been performed. Where available, recording of EEG to assess the efficacy of treatment is consistent with values and preferences of limiting sequels of neonatal seizures. However, the net benefits are context-specific. In resource-challenged health care centres where EEG is not available, response to treatment is best assessed by clinical observation.

- The purpose of recording EEG for prognosis determination is based upon the idea of maximizing infant potential through early intervention. While there may be enhanced accuracy in the prediction of long-term outcome by utilizing EEG, serial recordings would imply a cost to be borne both on families and health care systems for data that may not have immediate implications.

Recommendation(s)

- Where available, all clinical seizures in the neonatal period should be confirmed by electroencephalography (strong, context-specific recommendation).

- Electroencephalography should not be performed for the sole purpose of determining the etiology in neonates with clinical seizures (strong recommendation).

Question 9

What is the value of imaging of the cranium/head in diagnosis, evaluation of etiology, treatment, and prognosis of the newborn with seizures?

Summary of evidence – Values and benefits

Ultrasound (US). *One study (Malik et al., 2005) reported that in about 10% of infants with NS an abnormal finding was found on head US, while another study (Alcover-Bloch et al., 2004) reported 43% of infants with abnormal head US.*

Computed tomography (CT)/Magnetic Resonance Imaging (MRI). *One study reported that in term neonates with seizures MRI findings did not correlate with either clinical signs of perinatal distress or perinatal causes of cerebral injury (Rollins et al., 1994); similarly, another study noted that severity of seizures in newborns with perinatal asphyxia is independently associated with brain injury and is not limited to damage detectable by MRI (Miller et al., 2002).*

US vs. CT/MRI. *One retrospective study reported that about 43% of neonates with seizures had an abnormal head US, while only 31% had abnormal findings on CT and/or MRI (Rollins et al., 1994); another study (Mercuri et al., 1995) noted that 88% (14/16) of neonates with seizures had haemorrhage or ischaemia detected on MRI, with 11 of them detectable by US, and that MRI could detect ischaemic lesions earlier than US.*

- There are no data to support the use of neuroimaging in determining whether clinical or electrographic seizures are present. However, it can be a useful tool in the diagnosis of intracranial lesions that may be associated with NS.
- Each modality – US, CT or MRI – has its relative strengths and weakness in the diagnosis of various intracranial disorders; their conduct does not support any values or preferences when used in this way.
- These tests can be expensive and resource-consuming. In addition, the technology may be difficult to maintain and operate in low-resource areas.
- There are no data supporting the use of neuroimaging to determine the efficacy of AED treatment.
- There is low quality evidence that the findings of neuroimaging can be utilized as one of several factors in determining long-term outcome; the benefit to conduct these tests to assess prognosis is unclear, and related to the etiologic findings.

Recommendation(s)

- Radiological investigations (ultrasound, computed tomography and magnetic resonance imaging) of the cranium/head should not be performed to determine the presence or absence of clinical seizures or to evaluate the efficacy of treatment with antiepileptic drugs in neonates (strong recommendation).
- They may be performed as part of the comprehensive evaluation of the etiology of neonatal seizures or to determine prognosis in neonates with seizures (weak, context-specific recommendation).

Annexes

Annex 1: List of contributors

Guideline Development Group

In alphabetical order

Ramesh K. Agarwal
Associate Professor
WHO/CC for Training and Research in Newborn Care &
ICMR Centre for Advanced Research in Newborn Health
Neonatal Health Knowledge Centre (NHKC)
Division of Neonatology, Department of Paediatrics
All India Institute of Medical Sciences, New Delhi, India.

John Patrick T. Co
Director, Outpatient Quality and Safety, MassGeneral Hospital for Children
Director, Graduate Medical Education, Partners HealthCare
Assistant Professor of Paediatrics, Harvard Medical School
MGH Center for Child and Adolescent Health Research and Policy
Boston, MA, USA

J Helen Cross
Professor, The Prince of Wales's Chair of Childhood Epilepsy
Chair ILAE Commission for Paediatrics 2005-2009
UCL-Institute of Child Health
Great Ormond Street Hospital for Children & National Centre
for Young People with Epilepsy
Head of Neurosciences Unit
London, Great Britain

Maurizio Elia
Head of the WHO/CC for Training and Research on Neuroscience
Director of the Unit of Neurology and Neurophysiology
Department of Mental Retardation
IRCCS Associazione Oasi Maria SS. – ONLUS
Troina (EN) – Italy

Renzo Guerrini
Professor and Director
Clinic of Paediatric Neurology
Meyer University Hospital
Florence, Italy

Hans Hartmann
Consultant Pediatric Neurologist
Department of Pediatric Kidney, Liver and Metabolic Diseases
Hannover Medical School
Hannover, Germany

Nebojsa Jovic
Professor
Clinic of Neurology and Psychiatry for Children and Youth
Faculty of Medicine
Belgrade, Serbia

Angelina M. Kakooza
President, ILAE, Epilepsy Society Uganda (EPISOU)
Treasurer, ILAE, Commission on African Affairs.
Board Member, ILAE, Commission on Education.
Lecturer, Department of Paediatrics & Child Health
Makerere University College of Health Sciences
School of Medicine
Kampala, Uganda

Eli M. Mizrahi
Chair, Department of Neurology
Professor of Neurology and Pediatrics
Baylor College of Medicine
Houston, TX, USA

Emmanuel Raffo
Professor
Paediatric Neurology
Université de Lorraine - INSERM U 94
Hôpital d'Enfants - CHU de Nancy
Nancy, France

Jo Wilmshurst
Associate Professor
Department of Paediatric Neurology
Red Cross Children's Hospital
Cape Town, South Africa

Elizabeta Zisovska
Professor of Pediatrics
Chief of the Department of Neonatology, Gynecology & Obstetric Clinic
Skopje, Republic of Macedonia

WHO Secretariat

Rajiv Bahl
Medical Officer
Department of Maternal, Newborn, Child and Adolescent Health
World Health Organization
Geneva, Switzerland

Dr Tarun Dua
Medical Officer
Department of Mental Health and Substance Abuse
World Health Organization
Geneva, Switzerland

Other key contributors

José Manoel Bertolote
Professor, AISRAP
Griffith University, Australia
Associate Professor,
Faculdade de Medicina de Botucatu – UNESP
Botucatu, Brazil

Bernardo Dalla Bernardina
Professor
Unit of Child Neuropsychiatry
University of Verona
Verona, Italy

Hanneke de Boer
Global Campaign Against Epilepsy Coordinator
Stichting Epilepsie Instellingen Nederland (SEIN, WHO CC for Research, Training and Treatment in Epilepsy)
Senior Officer International Contacts
Hoofddorp, The Netherlands

Deborah Hirtz
Program Director, Office of Clinical Research
National Institute of Neurological Disorders and Stroke
National Institutes of Health
Rockville, MD, USA

Solomon L. Moshé
President, International League Against Epilepsy
Charles Frost Chair In Neurosurgery and Neurology
Professor of Neurology, Neuroscience & Pediatrics
Vice-Chair, Dept. of Neurology
Director, Pediatric Neurology,
Director, Clinical Neurophysiology
Albert Einstein College of Medicine
Bronx, NY, USA

M Jeeva Sankar
Medical Officer
Department of Maternal, Newborn, Child and Adolescent Health
World Health Organization
Geneva, Switzerland

Martin Weber
Medical Officer
Child and Adolescent Health and Development
WHO country office
Jakarta, Indonesia

Annex 2: GRADE profiles and summary of individual studies

Prevalence of various causes of neonatal seizures in different geographical regions of the world

TABLE 1

Study population	Study period	Hypoxic-ischaemic encephalopathy	Hypoglycaemia	Hypocalcaemia	CNS infection
Only full term neonates	**Until 1990**	Eriksson & Zetterström - 48% Rose & Lombroso - 13% Gunn & Cable - 83% *Range: 13 to 83%* *Median: 48%*	Eriksson & Zetterström - 6.5% Rose & Lombroso - 5% Gunn & Cable - NA *Range: 5 to 6.5%* *Median: 5.5%*	Eriksson & Zetterström - 2.6% Rose & Lombroso - 20% Gunn & Cable - 9% *Range: 2.6 to 20%* *Median: 9%*	Eriksson & Zetterström - 12% Rose & Lombroso - 9.5% Gunn & Cable – NA *Range: 9.5 to 12%* *Median: 10.3%*
	Since 1990	Lien et al.- 38% *Range: NA* *Median: 38%*	Lien et al. - NA	Lien et al. - NA	Lien et al. - 7.5% *Range: NA* *Median: 7.5%*
Mixed (full term and preterm neonates) or not known	**Until 1990**	Craig - NA Schulte - 54% Keen & Lee - 12,5% (+ICH) Combes et al. - 77% (+ICH) Rossiter et al. - NA Dennis - 44% (including hypoglycaemia and hypocalcaemia) Andre et al. - 56% McInerny & Schubert - 33% Langevin - 57% Ellison et al. - 24% Holden et al. - NA Ment et al. - 32% Goldberg - 30 to 41% Bergman et al. - 59% Zalneraitis - 74% Tudehope et al. - 40% *Range: 12.5% to 77%* *Median: 42.5%*	Craig - NA Schulte - NA Keen & Lee - 4% Combes et al. - NA Rossiter et al. - 13% Dennis - 12% Andre et al. - 1.4% McInerny & Schubert - 7% Langevin - NA Ellison et al. - NA Holden et al. - NA Ment et al. - NA Goldberg - 1 to 11% Bergman et al. - 5% Zalneraitis - NA Tudehope et al. - NA *Range: 1% to 13%* *Median: 6%*	Craig 0.5% Schulte - NA Keen & Lee - 42% Combes et al. - 10% Rossiter et al. - NA Dennis - 14% (pure) Andre et al. - 2.8% McInerny & Schubert - 30% Langevin - 43% Ellison et al. - 2% Holden et al. - NA Ment et al. - NA Goldberg - 4 to 6% Bergman et al. - 1.5% Zalneraitis - NA Tudehope et al. - NA *Range: 0.5% to 43%* *Median: 6%*	Craig - 6% Schulte - 7% Keen & Lee - 0.7% Combes et al. - 7% Rossiter et al. - 13% Dennis - NA Andre et al. - 24% McInerny & Schubert - 10% Langevin - NA Ellison et al. - 3% Holden et al. - 17% Ment et al. - 11% Goldberg - 4 to 5% Bergman et al. - 12% Zalneraitis - 13% Tudehope et al. - 11% *Range: 0.7% to 24%* *Median: 10%*
	Since 1990	Toet et al. - 80% Legido et al. - 35% Lanska & Lanska - 40% Ortibus et al. - 37% Ronen et al. - 40% Brunquell et al. - 49% Garcias da Silva et al. - 34% Bye et al. - 42% Idro et al. - 12% *Range: 12% to 80%* *Median: 40%*	Toet et al. - NA Legido et al. - NA Lanska & Lanska - NA Ortibus et al. - NA Ronen et al. - 13% Brunquell et al. - NA Garcias da Silva et al. - NA Bye et al. - 4% Idro et al. - NA *Range: 4% to 13%* *Median: 8.5%*	Toet et al. - NA Legido et al. - NA Lanska & Lanska - NA Ortibus et al. - NA Ronen et al. - 5% Brunquell et al. - NA Garcias da Silva et al. - NA Bye et al. - NA Idro et al. - 5%	Toet et al. - NA Legido et al. - 12.5% Lanska & Lanska - Ortibus et al. - 9% Ronen et al. - 8% Brunquell et al. - 2% Garcias da Silva et al. - 13% Bye et al. - 6% Idro et al. - 6% *Range: 2% to 13%* *Median: 8%*
Preterm neonates or low birth weight	**Until 1990**	Seay & Bray - 87% (birthweight<2,5kg) Watkins et al. - 40% *Range: 40% to 87%* *Median: 63.5 %*	Seay & Bray - NA Watkins et al. - 3% *Range: NA* *Median: 3%*	Seay & Bray - 3% Watkins et al. - 1.5% *Range: 1.5% to 3%* *Median: 2.3%*	Seay & Bray - 6% Watkins et al. - 5% *Range: 5% to 6%* *Median: 5.5%*
	Since 1990	---	---	---	---

Note. GRADE could not be applied to epidemiological data *NA= not available*

Summary of individual studies

Note. GRADE criteria could not be applied to epidemiological data

Prospective studies. *Ronen et al. (2007), Tekgul et al. (2006), Ortibus et al. (1996), Pisani et al. (2008b), Plouin et al. (1981), Dreyfus-Brisac et al. (1981) and Bye et al. (1997) conducted prospective cohort studies, noting an association between neonatal seizures and abnormal neurological outcome, morbidity, and mortality. Both Mizrahi & Kellaway (1987) and Rowe et al. (1985) noted that EEG characteristics can help determine etiology and outcomes. McBride et al. (2000) noted an association between the amount of electrographic seizure activity and subsequent mortality and morbidity in infants at risk for seizures and in infants with perinatal asphyxia. Similarly, Laroia et al. (1998) noted that a normal EEG in the neonatal period is associated with the absence of seizures within the first two years of life, with a sensitivity of 0.96 and specificity of 0.81. Kerr et al. (1990) found that EEGs can help predict persistence of seizures. Scarpa et al. (1983), Kumar et al. (2007) and Bye & Flanagan (1995) noted that use of EEG could help with anticonvulsant management, while Connell et al. (1989) showed mixed results to this regard. Murray et al. (2008) noted that only one third of neonates with electrographic seizures had clinical signs.*

Retrospective studies. *Khan et al. (2008), Pisani et al. (2008a) and Carrascosa et al. (1996) noted an association between abnormal EEG findings and neurological outcome, including developmental delay, epilepsy and death. Van Rooij et al. (2007) noted that duration, but not background pattern, was associated with neurodevelopmental outcome. Tharp et al. (1981) noted that using serial EEGs (also in the neonatal period) can help determine prognosis, including neurodevelopmental outcomes. Hosain et al. (2003) noted that EEG helped identify apnoeic seizures. Pezzani et al. (1986) noted that EEG on the first day of life can help assess the degree of brain injury. Radvanyi-Bouvet et al. (1985) noted that in premature infants EEG can be helpful in assessment and therapy of atypical seizures. Staudt (1990) noted a correlation between abnormal background activity and prognosis. Domenech-Martinez et al. (2003) noted that moderately to markedly abnormal background EEG activity had a high positive predictive value for abnormal outcomes and can be helpful in assessing response to therapy.*

Table 2

Study/Country	Design	Summary of study	Quality	Sample size	Comments
AMERICAS					
Khan et al., 2008, Brazil	Retrospective	Sequential EEG can better help predict neurological outcome (neurodevelopmental delay, epilepsy, death)	Low	58	This study was used to show the benefit of doing sequential EEGs, with the analysis looking for association between abnormal EEGs and outcomes.
Ronen et al., 2007, Canada	Prospective cohort	EEG can help predict neurological outcome	Low	82	This study was a long-term follow-up study with children who had seizures in the neonatal period, and looked for statistical association between abnormal EEGs and outcomes.
Tekgul et al., 2006, USA	Prospective	EEG is prognostic of neurodevelopmental outcome	Low	98	This was a short-term (1.5 years) follow-up study that tested for statistical association between abnormal EEGs and outcomes.
Ortibus et al., 1996, USA	Prospective	EEG is a predictor of neurodevelopmental outcome, but not postnatal seizures	Low	81	Neonates with seizures followed for 17 months (on average); analysis looked for association and multivariate models for predicting seizures and outcomes.
Hosain et al., 2003, USA	Retrospective	Continuous EEG helps diagnose apnoeic seizures	Low	10	Six patients had nonspecific findings consisting of multifocal interictal epileptiform activity with no event correlation. Continuous 24-72-hour EEG was performed in all patients to rule out apnoeic seizures. Ictal EEG showed high correlation with the apnoeic episodes, confirming the diagnosis of apnoeic seizures.
McBride et al., 2000, USA	Prospective	EEG can help predict mortality and morbidity	Moderate	68	Control group; the occurrence of ES was correlated with microcephaly ($p = 0.04$), severe CP ($p = 0.03$), and failure to thrive ($p = 0.03$). In the subgroup of infants with asphyxia, those with ES were more likely to die of neurologic causes ($p = 0.02$) and have microcephaly ($p = 0.05$) or severe CP ($p = 0.04$). Additionally, those with the greatest number of electrographic seizures were more likely to have these severe outcomes.
Laroia et al., 1998, USA	Retrospective and prospective, cohort	Normal/immature EEG predicts absence of seizures in the next 18-to-24 hours with 96% sensitivity and 81% specificity	Low	29	EEG done on at risk infants, none of them already had ever had a seizure.
Kerr et al., 1990, USA	Prospective cohort	EEG can help predict whether seizures continue; use of both short-term and ambulatory EEGs can result in some incremental benefit	Low	13	Thirteen neonates with seizures occurring after 7 days of age were evaluated with standard short-term EEG during the initial seizures and with ambulatory EEG when each infant was within 37-44 weeks of corrected age (i.e. gestational age plus chronologic age). Eight out of 13 standard EEGs, 10 out of 13 ambulatory EEGs, and 12 out of 13 with the combined use of both standard EEGs and ambulatory EEGs accurately predicted the occurrence of seizures at 3-4 months of corrected age. Results with standard EEG and ambulatory EEG did not produce significantly different outcomes. Combined analysis of standard EEG and ambulatory EEG produced significantly different results from those calculated when the two EEG types were analyzed independently ($Z = 3.98$, p = less than 0.001). Findings indicate that the use of both tests may improve the ability to predict continued seizure activity in infants with neonatal seizures when compared to the use of each measure separately. This study looked at testing strategies for predicting continuance of seizures, and NOT its usefulness in current management.
Mizrahi & Kellaway, 1987, USA	Prospective cohort	Study to characterize and classify neonatal seizures	Low	349	Study looked at association between EEG findings and clinical symptoms and outcomes.
Rowe et al., 1985, USA	Prospective cohort	EEG can help predict outcome	Low	74	Follow-up of children with a mean age of 33 months; looked for association between EEG findings and outcomes.
Tharp et al., 1981, USA	Retrospective cohort	EEG can help determine prognosis	Low	81	Premature infants; infants whose serial EEGs were normal during the neonatal period were usually normal at follow-up or suffered from minor sequelae (NPV: 100%). All children who had at least one markedly abnormal EEG suffered from some type of neurological sequelae or died. This study analyzed the value of serial EEGs.
Scher et al., 1993, USA	Retrospective	EEG can help confirm seizures	Low	92	This study mainly compared differing seizure characterization between term and pre-term infants.

EUROPE					
Pisani et al., 2008b, Italy	Prospective	Helpful in prognosis of developmental outcome	Low	38	Study looked for association of EEG findings with neurodevelopmental outcome.
Murray et al., 2008, Ireland	Prospective	Only one third of neonatal EEG seizures displays clinical manifestations; video EEG used for the study	Low	51	Only one-third of neonatal EEG seizures displays clinical signs on simultaneous video recordings. Moreover, two-thirds of these clinical manifestations are unrecognized, or misinterpreted by experienced neonatal staff. In the recognition and management of neonatal seizures clinical diagnosis alone is not enough.
Pisani et al., 2008a, Italy	Retrospective cohort, prospective follow-up	EEG can help predict neurological outcome	Low	51 pre-term infants	Severely abnormal background EEG activity (OR=8.298, 95% CI: 1.316-52.301, p=0.024) were independent predictors of abnormal outcome. Nine infants presented post-neonatal epilepsy. Severely abnormal cerebral ultrasound scans were predictive of epilepsy (OR=13.72, 95% CI: 1.959-96.149, p=0.008). This study used odds ratio to estimate differences in outcomes according to EEG results.
Van Rooij et al., 2007, Netherlands	Retrospective	EEG is the main predictor of neurodevelopmental outcome	Low	56	The duration, but not the background pattern, was correlated with neurodevelopmental outcome; this study looked for EEG characteristics that would help predict outcome, but did not look at the incremental benefit of doing EEG *vs.* not doing EEG.
Pezzani et al., 1986, Italy	Retrospective	EEG in the first day of life can help assess degree of cerebral injury	Low	80	Study characterized EEG findings associated with unfavourable outcome (death, major sequelae).
Radvanyi-Bouvet et al., 1985, France	Retrospective	EEG can be helpful in recognition of atypical seizures and assessment of the effectiveness of therapy	Low	50 premature	Cohort broken into subgroups according to gestational age at delivery→ small subgroups.
Domenech-Martinez et al., 2003, Spain	Retrospective	EEG is helpful in diagnosing and assessing response to treatment	Low	74	Infants with moderately and markedly abnormal EEGs background showed unfavourable outcomes in 72.2% PPV and 100% PPV of cases respectively, while only 15.4% (84.6% NPV) had normal or lightly abnormal EEGs background.
Carrascosa et al., 1996, Spain	Retrospective, cohort	EEG somewhat helpful to predict outcome, but cause of seizure and cerebral lesion most important factors	Low	25	I. Differences were found between the types of seizures presented (clonic, focal tonic, myoclonic, subtile with apnoea, no obvious seizure) and the prognosis, but no significant results. Neurological findings between seizures: those who showed no change in consciousness following the convulsion had a better prognosis than those showing changes. The difference was significant (P=0.03). Post-critic EEG pattern: those with normal or focal EEG were grouped together *vs.* those who showed multifocal alterations, presented with changes in the basic rhythm, were paroxysmal or of low voltage; the first type of EEG indicated the best prognosis (OR=12.0; IC 95%; 1.1-159.5; p=0.2). Radiodiagnosis: those with no changes on US or CT-MRI had better prognoses (p>0.001) than those with pathological ones. None had pathological sequelae (OR=0.0). II. Multivariant analysis: the final method only retained the variable "Radiodiagnosis", implying that the other variables lost significance when corrected for association with Radiodiagnosis ($p < 0.001$; OR = 0.0).
Staudt, 1990, Germany *(Article in German, abstract in English reviewed)*	Retrospective cohort	EEG can help predict prognosis	Low	29	A correlation could be shown between poor prognosis and suppression of background activity consisting in inactivity, burst-suppression pattern or moderate suppression. By contrast, a normal or mildly suppressed EEG correlated with good long-term prognosis. Paroxysmal discharges in the EEG were helpful in diagnosing seizures and also for prognosis of cerebral convulsions later on. US and EEG findings, especially mild intracranial haemorrhages and increased periventricular echogenicity, had less prognostic value. Thus study looked for correlation of EEG findings and outcomes.
Connell et al., 1989, England	Prospective cohort	Response to anticonvulsants not consistently seen on EEG	Low	31	Background EEG abnormality (as an index of associated cerebral dysfunction) was a guide to potential lack of response to anticonvulsant drugs; it was also predictive of subsequent clinical outcome irrespective of treatment.
Scarpa et al., 1983, Italy	Prospective cohort	EEG can help plan for anticonvulsant management; the duration of persistence of EEG abnormalities was the most important finding for planning the maintenance of anticonvulsant treatment and its discontinuation	Low	55	EEG used for extended period of time, consequently, this study was not so useful.

Plouin et al.,1981, France *(article in French, abstract in English reviewed)*	Prospective cohort	EEG can help determine prognosis	Low	43	Ninety percent had favourable outcome. In the cases with unfavourable evolution, the following criteria allowed for early poor prognosis: a very early onset of the seizures in the first or second day of life, the presence of tonic seizures and hypertony between seizures, duration of seizures longer than 4 days, EEG activity in the frequency of the alpha band during the seizures, a flat tracing after the seizures, very discontinuous activity between the seizures and, finally, the reappearance of seizures after a seizure-free interval.
Dreyfus-Brisac et al., 1981 France *(article in French, abstract in English reviewed)*	Prospective cohort	EEG can help determine prognosis	Low	121	The very poor prognosis of an abnormal EEG pattern of the premature newborn, i.e. an EEG lacking any pattern corresponding to any gestational age, is demonstrated in this study. Such EEGs of very poor prognosis were detected in 46 cases. They reveal the degree of severity of the cerebral lesions, EEG abnormalities and cerebral lesions varying with gestational age. This study confirmed the relatively mild severity of isolated convulsions as compared to status epilepticus.
SOUTHEAST ASIA					
Kumar et al., 2007, India *(full text article could not be retrieved)*	Prospective	Abnormal EEG were found in one-third of children with clinical seizures	Low	90	Abnormal EEGs were found in one-third of cases out of 60 EEGs done in 90 infants. 26.7% of infants with perinatal asphyxia had abnormal EEGs (8/30), while 60% with HIE-II had abnormal discharges; background activity was suppressed in 66.66% EEGs in infants with HIE-III.
WESTERN PACIFIC					
Bye et al., 1997, Australia	Prospective, cohort	EEG can help predict survival	Low	53	Abnormal findings from brain imaging studies and a number of independent electrographic seizure foci were correlated with some aspects of the outcomes at 1 year. Note that this study looked for association between findings and outcomes.
Bye & Flanagan, 1995, Australia	Prospective cohort	EEG is helpful in diagnosis	Low	32	Thirty-two patients had confirmed seizures. After administration of anticonvulsants, clinical observations identified seizures in a mean of 66% (*SD*=7.3%) of the cohort. A 60-min EEG after each stage of phenobarbital therapy would guarantee electrographic seizure capture in a mean of 76% (*SD*=10%) of the cohort. A 60-min EEG after addition of phenytoin would guarantee capture in 50% of cases. Conclusions: EEG would avoid misdiagnoses in most patients with ambiguous clinical signs. After anticonvulsant infusions, EEG adds substantial information to that obtained from clinical observations.
Bye & Flanagan 1995, Australia	Prospective cohort	EEG can help detect subclinical seizures and response to therapy	Low	32	There was evidence of reduced clinical features after sequential AED infusions.

Value of cranium/head imaging in the management of a newborn with seizures

Summary of individual studies

Note. GRADE criteria could not be applied to epidemiological data

Malik et al. (2005) noted that approximately 10% of neonates with seizures showed an abnormal finding on head ultrasound (US). Alcover-Bloch et al. (2004) noted retrospectively that approximately 43% of neonates with seizures had an abnormal head US, while 31% had abnormal findings on CT and/or MRI. Rollins et al. (1994) noted that in term neonates with seizures, MRI findings did not correlate with either clinical signs of perinatal distress or perinatal causes of cerebral injury, while Krishnamoorthy et al. (2000) found that MRI helped identify seizure etiology. Miller et al. (2002) reported the severity of seizures in newborns with perinatal asphyxia as being independently associated with brain injury and not limited to damage detectable by MRI. Keeney et al. (1991) noted that in neonates prospectively determined to be at risk for neurologic handicap, US detected 79% of lesions demonstrated by MRI, whereas only 41% were detected by CT. Mercuri et al. (1995) found that 88% (14/16) of neonates with seizures had haemorrhage or ischaemia noted on MRI, with 11 of these detectable by US, and that MRI could detect ischaemic lesions earlier than US.

TABLE 3

Study/Country	Design	Summary of study	Quality	Sample size	Comments
AMERICAS					
Rollins et al., 1994, USA	Prospective	MRI done in term neonates with seizures; presence or pattern of MRI findings does not appear to correlate with clinical signs of perinatal distress or presumed causes of perinatal cerebral injury	Low	15	Small sample size; based on MRI, five patients had focal ischaemic injury of the cerebral hemispheres and/or basal ganglia and brain stem. Six patients had diffuse cerebral oedema: of these, five had basal ganglia oedema; one had brain stem oedema. One patient had superior sagittal sinus thrombosis with venous infarcts. Three patients had normal MRI studies. There was no correlation between markers of perinatal distress, risk factors for seizures, and presence or pattern of MRI findings.
Miller et al., 2002, USA	Prospective	Structural damage detected by MRI does not completely account for brain injury caused by perinatal asphyxia	Low	90 (only 33 had seizures)	This study looked at correlation of seizures with lactate/choline levels in different parts of the brain.
Krishnamoorthy et al., 2000, USA	Prospective	CT and MRI done; short-term neurologic outcome correlated with the extent of injury seen on the initial diffusion-weighted imaging scans for all patients	Low	8	Infants followed for a mean of 17 months; head CT, conventional MRI and diffusion-weighted images were obtained. All patients showed increased lesion conspicuity and better definition of lesion extent on the diffusion-weighted images compared with the CT and T2-weighted MRI. Diffusion-weighted imaging is useful in the evaluation of acute ischaemic brain injury and seizure etiology in neonates.
Keeney et al., 1991, USA	Prospective	Not all children in the study had seizures; MRI	Low	100	The usefulness of this study is somewhat limited in that children were at risk for poor outcomes, not necessarily all had a history of seizures.
EASTERN MEDITERRANEAN					
Malik et al., 2005, Pakistan	Prospective	9.5% with intracranial bleed, 1.5% hydrocephalus, 1% with brain malformations	Low	200	US done in all patients, CT done in a few; this study aimed to identify the etiology of seizures in a cohort of patients; for this review, the relevance was that approximately 10% had a finding on head US.
EUROPE					
Alcover-Bloch et al., 2004, Spain *(article in Spanish, abstract in English reviewed)*	Retrospective	Head US was abnormal in 33 infants, CT and/or MRI abnormal in 24	Low	77	This study aimed to identify the etiology of seizures in a cohort of patients, a high percentage of them showed an abnormality on a radiographic study.
Maynard & Garrel, 1983, France *(article in French, abstract in English reviewed)*	Prospective	US or CT done	Low	20	Small sample size, described findings in 20 newborns that had seizures during the first days of life.
Mercuri et al., 1995, England	Prospective	US and MRI done, MRI supplement findings from US	Low	16	Fourteen of the infants had haemorrhagic or ischaemic lesions on MRI and these were detected by ultrasound scanning in 11. Early ultrasound scanning detected haemorrhagic lesions, although ischaemic lesions were often not detected until the end of the first week of life. Early MRS, however, was able to detect all the ischaemic lesions.
Rufo-Campos et al., 2000, Spain *(article in Spanish, abstract in English reviewed)*	Retrospective	Haemorrhages were the second most common etiology of seizures	Low	60	Study investigated 22 medical variables related to the clinical history, neurological examination, neuroimaging studies, EEG and drugs used. Abnormalities were found on the initial examination in 83.3% of the cases. Hypoxic-ischaemic syndrome was the commonest etiology, followed by haemorrhages, metabolic disorders, cardiopathies, malformations and infectious diseases.
SOUTH-EAST ASIA					
Kumar et al., 2007, India *(full text article could not be retrieved)*	Prospective	US done, relation to seizures not described in abstract	Low	90	-

First-line antiepileptic drug for treatment of neonatal seizures

Patients: neonates with seizures requiring treatment

Intervention (exposure): phenobarbital as the first-line drug

Control (unexposed): any other antiepileptic drug as the first-line medication

Table 5 - GRADE table

OUTCOME	No. of studies	Design	Limitations of studies				Precision	Consistency	Generalizability/ Directness	Very large effect or dose response gradient	Overall Quality of Evidence	Pooled effect size (95% CI) or range of effect sizes (where pooled effect size not possible to ascertain)
			Allocation concealment (the two groups comparable and low risk of reverse causality)	Blinding or other approaches to reduce measurement bias	Loss to follow-up (<20%)	Analysis Intention to treat; cluster adjusted if applicable (adjusted for confounding)						
Seizure control (during the initial hospital stay)	1	RCT (0)	Unclear (-0.5)	No (intervention/ observers were not blind) (-0.5)	Yes (0)	Yes (0)	Effect not significant, with wide CI (-1.0)	Single study (-1.0)	From developed country setting (-0.5)	Nil	VERY LOW (Total score = -3.5)	RR 0.97 (0.54, 1.72)

Included for GRADE

Study ID	Design	Study population	Allocation concealment (groups comparable and reverse causality unlikely)	Blinding (low risk of measurement bias)	<20% loss to follow-up	Intention to treat analysis (adjusted for most potential confounders)	Outcome measurement	Number (%) in intervention (exposed) group	Number (%) in control (unexposed) group	Effect (95% CI)	Limitations/ comments
Painter et al., 1999 USA	RCT	Neonates with EEG confirmed seizures	Unclear	No (neither intervention nor observers were blinded)	Yes	Yes	Control of electrical seizures	13/30 (43.5%) in infants who received phenobarbital as first-line drug	13/29 (45%) in infants who received phenytoin as first-line drug	RR 0.97 (0.54, 1.72)	Neonates whose seizures were not controlled by the assigned drug were then treated with both drugs

Observational studies without any control group (not considered for GRADE)

Study ID	Design	Study population	% with outcome	Directness	Limitations	Other comments
Alcover-Bloch et al., 2004	Retrospective observational study	Preterm and term neonates with seizures; N=258	81.8%	Limited (does not answer if phenobarbital is better than other AEDs)	Retrospective data from a single center	No control group
Bartha et al., 2007	Retrospective observational study	Preterm and term neonates with seizures; N=322	82.0%	Limited	Retrospective data	No control group
Nunes et al. ,2008	Prospective observational study	Preterm and term neonates with seizures; N=101	62.0%	Limited	-	No control group
Boylan et al., 2002	Observational study	Preterm and term neonates with seizures; N=14	28.5%	Limited	-	No control group
Boylan et al., 2004	Observational study	Preterm and term neonates with seizures; N=22	50.0%	Limited	-	No control group

Table 6 - GRADE table

OUTCOME	N. of studies	Design	Limitations of studies				Precision	Consistency	Generalizability/ Directness	Very Large effect or dose response gradient	Overall Quality of Evidence	Pooled effect size (95% CI) or range of effect sizes (where pooled effect size not possible to ascertain)
			Allocation concealment (the two groups comparable and low risk of reverse causality)	Blinding or other approaches to reduce measurement bias	Loss to follow-up (<20%)	Analysis intention to treat; cluster adjusted if applicable (adjusted for confounding)						
Benzodiazepines (I) *vs.* Phenytoin (C)												
Seizure control (during the initial hospital stay)	1	Observational (-1.0)	No (-0.5)	Unclear (-0.5)	Yes (0)	No (-0.5)	Effect significant; lower limit of CI meaningful (0)	Single study (-1.0)	From developed country setting (-0.5)	Nil	VERY LOW (Total score = - 4.0)	RR 2.13 (1.48, 3.08)
Normal neuro-development	1	Observational (-1.0)	No (-0.5)	Unclear (-0.5)	Yes (0)	No (-0.5)	Effect not significant, with wide CI (-1.0)	Single study (-1.0)	From developed country setting (-0.5)	Nil	VERY LOW (Total score = - 5.0)	RR 1.15 (0.62, 2.14)
Lidocaine (I) *vs.* Benzodiazepines (C)												
Seizure control	2 (1 RCT and 1 observational)	Majority of evidence from observational (-1.0)	Unclear in both studies (-0.5)	Unclear in both studies (-0.5)	Yes in both studies (0)	Majority of evidence from the study with "No" (-0.5)	Pooled effect not significant, with wide CI (-1.0)	Both studies in the same direction (0)	Both from developed country settings (-0.5)	Nil	VERY LOW (Total score = - 4.0)	RR 1.78 (0.90, 3.52)
Normal neuro-development	2 (1 RCT and 1 observational)	Majority of evidence from observational (-1.0)	Unclear in both studies (-0.5)	Unclear in both studies (-0.5)	Yes in both studies (0)	Majority of evidence from the study with "No" (-0.5)	Pooled effect not significant, with wide CI (-1.0)	Only 2 studies, both in opposite direction (-1.0)	Both from developed country settings (-0.5)	Nil	VERY LOW (Total score = - 5.0)	RR 1.20 (0.36, 3.96)

1. BENZODIAZEPINES VS. PHENYTOIN

OUTCOME A): SEIZURE CONTROL (BOTH CLINICAL AND ELECTROCLINICAL)

Included for GRADE

Study ID	Design	Study population	Allocation concealment (groups comparable and reverse causality unlikely)	Blinding (low risk of measurement bias)	<20% loss to follow-up	Intention to treat analysis (adjusted for most potential confounders)	Outcome measurement	Number (%) in intervention (exposed) group	Number (%) in control (unexposed) group	Effect (95% CI)	Limitations/ comments
Castro Conde et al., 2005, Spain	Observational	Term neonates who have effect size even after maximal dose of phenobarbital	No (majority of controls were from a historical cohort – groups not comparable)	Unclear (no information on blinding of observers)	Yes	No	Favorable response to treatment (based on EEG criteria)	9/9 (100%) in infants who received midazolam as second-line agent	17/36 (47%) in infants who received phenytoin as second-line agent	RR 2.13 (1.48, 3.08)	Favorable response defined as no more than 2 ESs of <30 seconds duration per/h recording multiple doses of midazolam but only 1 dose of phenytoin

Observational studies without any control group, i.e. only benzodiazepine treatment (not considered for GRADE)

Study ID	Design	Study population	Number (%) with outcome	Directness	Limitations	Other comments
van Leuven et al., 2004	Observational study	Term neonates with HIE treated with midazolam	11/15 (73%)	Limited	-	No control group
Hu et al., 2003	Observational study	Neonates treated with midazolam	32/32 (100%)	Limited	-	No control group
Sheth et al., 1996	Observational study	Term and preterm neonates treated with midazolam	6/6 (100%)	Limited	-	No control group
Maytal et al., 1991	Observational study	Term and preterm neonates treated with lorazepam	6/7 (86%)	Limited	-	No control group

OUTCOME B): NORMAL NEURODEVELOPMENT

Study ID	Design	Study population	Allocation concealment (groups comparable and reverse causality unlikely)	Blinding (low risk of measure-ment bias)	<20% loss to follow-up	Intention to treat analysis (adjusted for most potential confounders)	Outcome measurement	Number (%) in intervention (exposed) group	Number (%) in control (unexposed) group	Effect (95% CI)	Limitations
Castro Conde et al., 2005, Spain	Observational	Term neonates who have electrical seizures even after maximal dose of phenobatbital	No (majority of controls were from a historical cohort – groups not comparable)	Unclear (no information on blinding of observers)	Yes	No	Normal neuro-development at 1 year	7/9 (78%) in infants who received midazolam as second-line agent	15/36 (42%) in infants who received phenytoin as second-line agent	RR 1.15 (0.62, 2.14)	

Summary tables of individual studies

Patients: neonates with seizures that are not controlled by the first-line treatment (predominantly pheno-barbital)

Intervention (exposure): benzodi-azepines

Control (unexposed): phenytoin

Patients: neonates with seizures that cannot be controlled by using the first-line treatment (predominantly phenobarbital)

Intervention (exposure): lidocaine (lignocaine)

Control (unexposed): benzodiazepines

2. LIDOCAINE VS. BENZODIAZEPINES

OUTCOME A): SEIZURE CONTROL (BOTH CLINICAL AND ELECTROCLINICAL)

Included for GRADE											
Study ID	**Design**	**Study population**	**Allocation concealment (groups comparable and reverse causality unlikely)**	**Blinding (low risk of measurement bias)**	**<20% loss to follow-up**	**Intention to treat analysis (adjusted for most potential confounders)**	**Outcome measurement**	**Number (%) in intervention (exposed) group**	**Number (%) in control (unexposed) group**	**Effect (95% CI)**	**Limitations/ comments**
Boylan et al., 2004 UK	RCT* (Weight = 13.0%)	Term neonates who have electrical seizures even after maximal dose of phenobarbital	Unclear	No	Yes	Yes	Control of electrical seizures	3/5 (60%) in neonates who received lignocaine as second-line drug	0/3 in neonates who received midazolam as second-line drug	RR 4.67 (0.32, 68.0)	Clonazepam was used in those infants whose parents refused to give consent (in the RCT, authors compared lignocaine and midazolam)
									0/3 in neonates who received clonazepam as second-line drug	RR 4.67 (0.32, 68.0)	Favorable response defined as no more than 2 electrical seizures of <30 sec duration per hour recording
Shany et al., 2007 Israel	Retro-spective chart review (Weight= 87.0%)	Infants born at or after 36 weeks of gestation with HIE and seizures even after first-line treatment with phenobarbital and diazepam	Unclear (no information on how the second-line agent was chosen)	Unclear (retrieved from the files)	Yes	No	Control of clinical and electrical seizures	17/22 (77%)	4/8 (50%)	RR 1.54 (0.74, 3.20)	

* *Infants who received clonazepam were not randomized (see* Limitations/comments *above)*

Observational studies without any control group, i.e. only benzodiazepine treatment (not considered for GRADE)						
Study ID	Design	Study population	Number (%) with outcome	Directness	Limitations	Other comments
Rey et al., 1990	Observational study	Term and preterm neonates treated with lidocaine; N=13	11/13 (85%)	Limited (does not answer if midazolam is better than phenytoin)	-	No control group
Hellstrom- Westas et al., 1988	Observational study	Neonates treated with lidocaine; N=46	42/46 (92%)	Limited	-	No control group

OUTCOME B): NORMAL NEURODEVELOPMENT

Study ID	Design	Study population	Allocation concealment (groups comparable and reverse causality unlikely)	Blinding (low risk of measurement bias)	<20% loss to follow-up	Intention to treat analysis (adjusted for most potential confounders)	Outcome measurement	Number (%) in intervention (exposed) group	Number (%) in control (unexposed) group	Effect (95% CI)	Limitations/ comments
Boylan et al., 2004 UK	RCT (Weight = 15.8%)	Term neonates who have ES even after maximal dose of phenobarbital	Unclear	No	Yes	Yes	Normal neuro-development	0/5 in neonates who received lignocaine as second-line drug	1/3 (33.3%) in neonates who received midazolam as second-line drug	RR 0.22 (0.01, 4.20)	
Shany et al., 2007 Israel	Retrospective chart review (Weight = 84.2%)	Infants born at or after 36 weeks of gestation with HIE and seizures even after first-line treatment with phenobarbital and diazepam	Unclear) (no information on how the second-line agent was chosen)	Unclear (retrieved from the files)	Yes	No	Normal neuro-development	9/22 (41%)	2/8 (25%)	RR 1.64 (0.44, 6.01)	

When to stop antiepileptic drugs in neonates with seizures?

Patients: neonates with seizures that are not controlled by the first-line treatment (predominantly phenobarbital)

Intervention (exposure): stopping antiepileptic drugs (at discharge)

Control (unexposed): continuing antiepileptic drugs after discharge from the hospital

Table 7 - GRADE table

OUTCOME	No. of studies	Design	Limitations of studies				Precision	Consistency	Generalizability/ Directness	Very large effect or dose response gradient	Overall Quality of Evidence	Pooled effect size (95% CI) OR range of effect sizes (where pooled effect size not possible to ascertain)
			Allocation concealment (the two groups comparable and low risk of reverse causality)	Blinding or other approaches to reduce measurement bias	Loss to follow-up (<20%)	Analysis intention to treat; cluster adjusted if applicable (adjusted for confounding)						
Seizure recurrence *(about up to 5 yrs of age in one study)*	3	All observational (-1.0)	Majority of evidence from studies with "No" (-0.5)	Majority of evidence from studies with "Yes" (0)	Majority of evidence from studies with "Yes" (0)	Majority of evidence from studies with "No" (-0.5)	Pooled effect significant but upper limit of CI in the 'null' range (-0.5)	All studies in the same direction (0)	All from developed country settings (-0.5)	Nil	VERY LOW (Total score = -3.0)	RR 0.66 (0.47, 0.93)
Epilepsy later in life *(about up to 5 yrs of age)*	1	Observational (-1.0)	Unclear (-0.5)	Yes (0)	Yes (0)	No (-0.5)	Effect not significant, with wide CI (-1.0)	Single study (-1.0)	From developed country setting (-0.5)	Nil	VERY LOW (Total score = -4.5)	RR 0.54 (0.25, 1.19)
Cerebral palsy *(about up to 5 yrs of age)*	1	Observational (-1.0)	Unclear (-0.5)	Yes (0)	Yes (0)	No (-0.5)	Effect not significant, with wide CI (-1.0)	Single study (-1.0)	From developed country setting (-0.5)	Nil	VERY LOW (Total score = -4.5)	RR 0.63 (0.31, 1.27)
Developmental delay *(about up to 5 yrs of age)*	1	Observational (-1.0)	Unclear (-0.5)	Yes (0)	Yes (0)	No (-0.5)	Effect not significant, with wide CI (-1.0)	Single study (-1.0)	From developed country setting (-0.5)	Nil	VERY LOW (Total score = -4.5)	RR 0.91 (0.64, 1.29)

OUTCOME A): RECURRENCE OF SEIZURES AFTER DISCHARGE

Study ID	Design	Study population	Allocation concealment (groups comparable and reverse causality unlikely)	Blinding (low risk of measurement bias)	<20% loss to follow-up	Intention to treat analysis (adjusted for most potential confounders)	Outcome measure-ment	Number (%) in intervention (exposed) group	Number (%) in control (unexposed) group	Effect (95% CI)	Limitations
Guillet & Kwon, 2007, USA	Observational	Gestation ≥34 weeks and onset of seizures within 5 days of birth and resolution within 7 days of onset of seizures	Unclear (risk of reverse causality cannot be ruled out)	Yes (data obtained from charts)	Yes	No	Seizure recurrence (after discharge)	22/99 (22.2%) in infants who were discharged home without anticonvulsants	10/33 (30.3%) in infants who were discharged home with phenobarbital	RR 0.73 (0.39, 1.38)	Retrospective chart review; decision to continue AED to the discretion of physicians
Bartha et al., 2007, USA	Observational	Infants with admission/ discharge diagnosis of NS	No (groups not comparable)	Yes (data retrieved from charts)	Yes <20% loss to follow-up	No	Need for second anticonvulsant (for continuing seizures)	20/78 (25.6%) in infants who were discharged home without anticonvulsants	110/298 (36.9%) in infants who were discharged home with phenobarbital	RR 0.69 (0.46, 1.04)	Neonates who were continued on AED had either clinical or electrical seizures at discharge
Hellstrom-Westas et al., 1988, Sweden	Observational						Seizure recurrence	2/34 (5.9%)	1/2 (50%)	RR 0.12 (0.02, 0.81)	

OUTCOME B): EPILEPSY IN LATER LIFE

Study ID	Design	Study population	Allocation concealment (groups comparable and reverse causality unlikely)	Blinding (low risk of measurement bias)	<20% loss to follow-up	Intention to treat analysis (adjusted for most potential confounders)	Outcome measurement	Number (%) in intervention (exposed) group	Number (%) in control (unexposed) group	Effect (95% CI)	Limitations
Guillet & Kwon, 2007 USA	Observational	Gestation ≥34 weeks and onset of seizures within 5 days of birth and resolution within 7 days of onset of seizures	Unclear (risk of reverse causality cannot be ruled out)	Yes (data obtained from charts)	Yes	No	Epilepsy until a mean age of about 5 years	13/99 (13.1%) in infants who were discharged home without anticonvulsants	8/33 (24.2%) in infants who were discharged home with phenobarbital	RR 0.54 (0.25, 1.19)	Retrospective chart review; decision to continue AED to the discretion of physicians

OUTCOME C): CEREBRAL PALSY

Study ID	Design	Study population	Allocation concealment (groups comparable and reverse causality unlikely)	Blinding (low risk of measurement bias)	<20% loss to follow-up	Intention to treat analysis (adjusted for most potential confounders)	Outcome measurement	Number (%) in intervention (exposed) group	Number (%) in control (unexposed) group	Effect (95% CI)	Limitations
Guillet & Kwon, 2007 USA	Observational	Gestation ≥34 weeks and onset of seizures within 5 days of birth and resolution within 7 days of onset of seizures	Unclear (risk of reverse causality cannot be ruled out)	Yes (data obtained from charts)	Yes	No	Cerebral palsy	17/99 (17.2%) in infants who were discharged home without anticonvulsants	9/33 (27.3%) in infants who were discharged home with phenobarbital	RR 0.63 (0.31, 1.27)	Retrospective chart review; decision to continue AED to the discretion of physicians

OUTCOME D): DEVELOPMENTAL DELAY

Study ID	Design	Study population	Allocation concealment (groups comparable and reverse causality unlikely)	Blinding (low risk of measurement bias)	<20% loss to follow-up	Intention to treat analysis (adjusted for most potential confounders)	Outcome measurement	Number (%) in intervention (exposed) group	Number (%) in control (unexposed) group	Effect (95% CI)	Limitations
Guillet & Kwon,2007 USA	Observational	Gestation ≥34 weeks and onset of seizures within 5 days of birth and resolution within 7 days of onset of seizures	Unclear (risk of reverse causality cannot be ruled out)	Yes (data obtained from charts)	Yes	No	Developmental delay	52/99 (52.5%) in infants who were discharged home without anticonvulsants	19/33 (57.6%) in infants who were discharged home with phenobarbital	RR 0.91 (0.64, 1.29)	Retrospective chart review; decision to continue AED to the discretion of physicians

How to stop antiepileptic drugs in neonates with seizures?

We did not identify any studies – either RCTs or observational – that compared different regimens of stopping AEDs.

Prophylactic treatment with phenobarbital in neonates with hypoxic-ischaemic encephalopathy

Patients: neonates with hypoxic-ischaemic encephalopathy (but yet to develop seizures)

Intervention (exposure): prophylactic treatment with phenobarbital or other antiepileptic drugs

Control (unexposed): no prophylaxis

Table 8 - GRADE table

OUTCOME	No. of studies	Design	Limitations of studies				Precision	Consistency	Generalizability/ Directness	Very large effect or dose response gradient	Overall Quality of Evidence	Pooled effect size (95% CI) OR range of effect sizes (where pooled effect size not possible to ascertain)
			Allocation concealment (the two groups comparable and low risk of reverse causality)	Blinding or other approaches to reduce measurement bias	Loss to follow-up (<20%)	Analysis intention to treat; cluster adjusted if applicable (adjusted for confounding)						
Mortality *(during initial hospital stay)*	2 (1 RCT and 1 observ-ational)	Majority of evidence from observ-ational study (-1.0)	Majority of evidence from studies with "No" (-0.5)	Yes in both studies (0)	Majority of evidence from studies with "Yes" (0)	No (-0.5)	Pooled effect not significant, with wide CI (-1.0)	Both studies in the same direction (0)	Both studies from developing country settings (0)		VERY LOW (Total score = -3.0)	RR 1.80 (0.78, 4.19)
Abnormal neurological outcome *(at discharge in 1 study, at 3 years in the other)*	2	RCTs (0)	Yes in both studies (0)	Majority of evidence from studies with "Yes" (0)	No for both studies (-0.5)	No for both studies (-0.5)	Pooled effect significant and lower limit of CI meaningful (0)	Only 2 studies, ES of both in the same direction (-0.5)	Majority of evidence from the study in developing country settings (0)		MODERATE (Total score = -1.5)	RR 0.44 (0.24, 0.79)
Incidence of seizures *(in the initial hospital stay)*	4 (3 RCTs and 1 observ-ational)	Majority of evidence from RCTs (0)	Majority of evidence from studies with "Yes" (0)	Majority of evidence from studies with "No" (-0.5)	Majority of evidence from studies with "No" (-0.5)	Majority of evidence from studies with "No" (-0.5)	Pooled effect not significant, with wide CI (-1.0)	ES of studies with <75% of total weight in the same direction as pooled effect (-1.0)	Majority of evidence from studies in developing country settings (0)		VERY LOW (Total score = -3.5)	RR 0.84 (0.34, 2.09) Random-effects model

OUTCOME A): MORTALITY

Study ID	Design	Study population	Allocation concealment (groups comparable and reverse causality unlikely)	Blinding (low risk of measurement bias)	<20% loss to follow-up	Intention to treat analysis (adjusted for most potential confounders)	Outcome measurement	Number (%) in intervention (exposed) group	Number (%) in control (unexposed) group	Effect (95% CI)	Limitations
Singh et al., 2005 India	RCT (Weight = 41.6%)	Gestation ≥34 weeks with low Apgar, fetal distress and features of HIE the first 6 hours after birth	Yes	Yes (no information but "hard" outcome)	No (25% loss)	No (post-randomization exclusions)	Until discharge	5/25 (20%) in infants who received intravenous phenobarbital at 20 mg/kg	3/20 (15%) in infants who did not receive any prophylaxis	RR 1.33 (0.36, 4.92)	-
Ajayi et al., 1998 Nigeria	Retrospective chart review (Weight = 58.4%)	Term neonates with Apgar scores ≤5 at one and five minutes	No (higher number of infants in exposed group had low Apgar scores; risk of reverse causality cannot be ruled out entirely)	Yes (from the records)	Yes	No (only partially adjusted)	Until discharge	7/57 (12%) in infants who received intravenous phenobarbital at 10 mg/kg	5/91 (5.5%) in infants who did not receive any prophylaxis	RR 2.24 (0.74, 6.71)	The 2 groups of infants were managed by 2 different consultants (to give prophylaxis or not decided by the consultant); used a smaller dose of phenobarbital

OUTCOME B): ABNORMAL NEUROLOGICAL OUTCOME

Study ID	Design	Study population	Allocation concealment (groups comparable and reverse causality unlikely)	Blinding (low risk of measurement bias)	<20% loss to follow-up	Intention to treat analysis (adjusted for most potential confounders)	Outcome measurement	Number (%) in intervention (exposed) group	Number (%) in control (unexposed) group	Effect (95% CI)	Limitations
Singh et al., 2005 India	RCT (Weight = 52.5%)	Gestation ≥34 weeks with low Apgar, fetal distress and features of HIE the first 6 hours after birth	Yes	Yes (no blind intervention; blind observers)	No (25% loss to follow-up)	No (post-randomization exclusions)	Abnormal neurological outcome at discharge	6/20 (30%) in infants who received intravenous phenobarbital at 20 mg/kg	9/17 (53%) in infants who did not receive any prophylaxis	RR 0.56 (0.25, 1.28)	No significant difference in the outcome also at 3 months (RR 0.36, CI 0.11, 1.2)
Hall et al., 1998 USA	RCT (Weight = 47.5%)	Term or post-term neonates with severe birth asphyxia	Yes	Unclear (no blind intervention; no information on blinding of observers)	No (22.5% loss to follow-up)	No (post-randomization exclusions)	Abnormal neurological outcome at 3 years	4/15 (27%) in infants who received intravenous phenobarbital at 40 mg/kg	13/16 (81%) in infants who did not receive any prophylaxis	RR 0.33 (0.14, 0.78)	The effect of prophylactic treatment was significant even after stepwise logistic regression (only P values given)

OUTCOME C): INCIDENCE OF SEIZURES DURING INITIAL HOSPITAL STAY

Study ID	Design	Study population	Allocation concealment (groups comparable and reverse causality unlikely)	Blinding (low risk of measurement bias)	<20% loss to follow-up	Intention to treat analysis (adjusted for most potential confounders)	Outcome measurement	Number (%) in intervention (exposed) group	Number (%) in control (unexposed) group	Effect (95% CI)	Limitations
Singh et al., 2005 India	RCT (Weight = 19.2%)	Gestation ≥34 weeks with low Apgar, fetal distress and features of HIE the first 6 hours after birth	Yes	No (no blind intervention and outcome not "hard")	No (25% loss)	No (post-randomization exclusions)	Seizures during initial stay	2/25 (8%) in infants who received intravenous phenobarbital at 20 mg/kg	8/20 (40%) in infants who did not receive any prophylaxis	RR 0.20 (0.05, 0.84)	
Vargas-Origel et al., 2004 Mexico	RCT (Weight = 20.4%)						Seizures during initial stay	4/37 (10.8%) in infants who received intravenous phenobarbital at 40 mg/kg	4/36 (11.1%) in infants who did not receive any prophylaxis	RR 0.97 (0.26, 3.60)	
Hall et al., 1998 USA	RCT (Weight = 32.7%)	Term or post-term neonates with severe birth asphyxia	Yes	Unclear (no blind intervention; no information on blinding of observers)	No (22.5% loss)	No (post-randomization exclusions)	Seizures during initial stay	9/15 (60%) in infants who received intravenous phenobarbital at 40 mg/kg	14/16 (87.5%) in infants who did not receive any prophylaxis	RR 0.69 (0.44, 1.08)	
Ajayi et al., 1998 Nigeria	Retro-spective chart review (Weight = 27.7%)	Term neonates with Apgar scores ≤5 at one and five minutes	No (higher number of infants in exposed group had low Apgar scores)	Yes (from the records)	Yes	No (only partially adjusted)	Until discharge	13/57 (23%) in infants who received intravenous phenobarbital at 10 mg/kg	8/91 (9%) in infants who did not receive any prophylaxis	RR 2.59 (1.15, 5.87) Adjusted OR 1.8 (0.7, 4.7)	The 2 groups of infants were managed by 2 different consultants; used a smaller dose of phenobarbital

Summary of evidence

Empirical treatment of hypoglycaemia

Hypoglycaemia can be deleterious and is associated with sequelae including epilepsy (Caraballo et al., 2004). A risk/benefit analysis of empirical treatment is not available. Possible risks include worsening of hyperglycaemia in neonates with HIE, which is the most frequent etiological factor associated with NS. Since blood glucose can easily be measured at low cost, this should be performed before treatment.

Empirical treatment of hypocalcaemia

The incidence/prevalence of hypocalcaemia in neonates with seizures is highly variable. Studies that have found a very high incidence were published in the 1970s (Keen et al., 1973; Langevin,1974). With better nutritional management, the incidence of hypocalcaemia may ever since have declined. However, the data available are not sufficient to prove this assumption. Measurement of blood calcium is possible in hospital settings without time delay though less easily available than measurement of blood sugar. When given intravenously, calcium may cause significant harm, i.e. asystoly or skin necrosis. The benefit *vs.* harm ratio of empirical treatment of hypocalcaemia before laboratory tests cannot be assessed.

Empirical antibiotic treatment

Data on different etiologies of neonatal seizures are highly inconsistent. There is not sufficient evidence to describe regional differences. However, in the only available study from an African country, Idro and colleagues recently found a very high incidence of bacterial infections in neonates with seizures admitted at a hospital in Kenya (Idro et al., 2008). This study may be biased because only neonates referring to the hospital were included. Authors do not state whether the neonates showed other clinical signs of infection and give no information about laboratory tests performed. Since oral treatment of neonatal sepsis or pyogenic meningitis is not considered as a standard therapy, empirical treatment implies intravenous therapy.

Empirical antiviral treatment

Congenital herpes simplex virus infection is a rare cause of NS. In their population-based case-control study, Hall et al. found an increased odds ratio of 2.92 for a history of vaginal delivery/maternal herpes simplex infection in neonates presenting with seizures within the first 72 hours of life (Hall et al., 2006). The authors do not state whether the neonates showed other clinical signs of infection. Since oral treatment of congenital herpes simplex virus infection is not considered as a standard therapy, empirical treatment implies intravenous therapy. A benefit *vs.* harm ratio cannot be assessed due to paucity of data.

Empirical pyridoxine treatment

Pyridoxine dependent epilepsy is a rare disease with an incidence of definite and probable cases of 1:396,000 (Been et al., 2005) compared to the overall incidence of NS between 1:71 to 1:1000. Other treatable neonatal epileptic encephalopathies with metabolic causes, such as pyridoxal-phosphate dependent epilepsy probably are even less frequent; only case reports and small series of patients have been published and an incidence cannot be calculated. Diagnosis of pyridoxine dependent epilepsy can be established clinically by a positive response to treatment with pyridoxine. Failure to diagnose this condition may have deleterious effects on affected neonates, but delay in treatment of other underlying etiologies may also cause harm. A benefit *vs.* harm ratio cannot be calculated.

Empirical treatment for hypoglycaemia, hypocalcaemia and infections with seizures

No controlled trials were identified and therefore GRADE could not be applied

Predicting the prognosis in neonates with seizures

Outcome: recurrence of seizures

Patients: neonates with seizures that are controlled by one or more antiepileptic drugs

Exposed group: infants with the said predictor in neonatal period/at discharge

Unexposed group: infants with abnormal neurological examination in neonatal period/at discharge

Table 9 - *Outcome a) recurrence of seizures*

Predictor 1: normal neurological examination in neonatal period/at discharge

Study ID	Design	Outcome	Number (%) in exposed group	Number (%) in control group	Effect (95% CI)	Directness	Limitations
Labrecque et al., 1984	Retrospective cohort	Seizure recurrence	2/43 (4.6%)	4/7(57.1%)	RR 0.08 (0.02 to 0.36)	Yes	Observational study
Brod et al., 1988	Retrospective cohort	Seizure recurrence	0/10	5/14 (35.7%)	RR 0.12 (0.01, 2.02)	Yes	Observational study
Gherpelli et al., 1992	Retrospective cohort	Seizure recurrence	0/11	7/12 (58.3%)	RR 0.07 (0, 1.36)	Yes	Observational study

Predictor 2: normal EEG in neonatal period/at discharge

Study ID	Design	Outcome	Number (%) in exposed group	Number (%) in control group	Effect (95% CI)	Directness	Limitations
Scarpa et al., 1983	Retrospective cohort	Seizure recurrence	4/43	8/8	RR 0.09 (0.04 to 0.24)	Yes	Observational study
Brod et al ., 1988	Retrospective cohort	Seizure recurrence	4/22	5/8	RR 0.29 (0.10 to 0.82)	Yes	Observational study
Brod et al., 1988	Retrospective cohort	Seizure recurrence	1/10	4/5	RR 0.13 (0.02 to 0.84))	Yes	Observational study
Clancy & Legido, 1991	Retrospective cohort	Seizure recurrence	2/8	13/19	RR 0.37 (0.11 to 1.26)	Yes	Observational study
Gherpelli et al., 1992	Retrospective cohort	Seizure recurrence	2/18	5/5	RR 0.11 (0.03 to 0.41)	Yes	Observational study

Predictor 3: normal cranial US in neonatal period/at discharge

Study ID	Design	Outcome	Number (%) in exposed group	Number (%) in control group	Effect (95% CI)	Directness	Limitations
Gherpelli et al., 1992	Retrospective cohort	Seizure recurrence	1/11	4/7	RR 0.16 (0.02 to 1.15)	Yes	Observational study

Predictor 4: status of multiple parameters (electroencephalography, neurological examination, neuroimaging, resolution of underlying condition, etc.) in neonatal period/at discharge

Study ID	Design	Outcome	Number (%) in exposed group	Number (%) in control group	Effect (95% CI)	Directness	Limitations
Gherpelli et al., 1992	Retrospective cohort	Seizure recurrence	1/11	4/7	RR 0.16 (0.02 to 1.15)	Yes	Observational study

OUTCOME B): OTHER OUTCOMES

Study	Methods	Predictor	Outcome	Design of study	Consistency	Directness	Limitations of study
Legido et al., 1991	Cohort, retrospective study N=40	Developmental assessment	Favourable outcome (normal development), unfavourable (death, epilepsy, developmental delay, cerebral palsy); follow-up ranged from 5 to 56 months	moderate	Inconsistent in terms of brain maturity	limited	Sensitivity of clinical recognition of NS was low (21%); size of subgroups with different etiologies is small to have statistical power
Ortibus et al., 1996	Cohort study, prospective analysis N=81	EEG monitoring (ictal, interictal records, background activity, negative and positive sharp waves, interictal neurological examination: normal, moderately abnormal, severely abnormal; neuroimaging studies (cranial US, CT, MRI); developmental assessment	Long term outcome: favourable, unfavourable (normal, mildly abnormal, severely abnormal); development of post-neonatal epilepsy	good	good	useful	No video-EEG recordings were performed; lack of monitoring may result in missed neonates with brief or rare seizures
Temple et al., 1995	Cohort study, retrospective analysis N=22	Neuropsychological assessment of intelligence, spelling, memory, social adjustment applied at age 6 and ages 18-19 years	Long term cognitive outcome: cognitive decline (specific learning disabilities), normal development	moderate	moderate		No details relating to severity, type and EEG confirmation of NS
Boylan et al., 1999	Cohort study, prospective analysis N=24	Video-EEG 17 pts with electrographic/clinical seizures, 7 pts clinical-only seizures	Background EEG abnormal in all but one, revealed poor neurodevelopmental outcome	moderate	Inconsistency in terms of brain maturity and in type of seizures	moderate	It is not clear that clinical seizures alone were of epileptic nature; electrographic seizures alone were not separately studied
McBride et al., 2000	Observational prospective study with control group N=68	Outcome cohort of neonates with and without neonatal seizures based on identification of electrographic seizures	Amount of electrographic seizure activity correlated with subsequent mortality and morbidity	good	good	Identified need to treat all seizures with quite good evidence to improve outcome	Need randomized blinded comparison study to assess this

Study	Methods	Predictor	Outcome	Design of study	Consistency	Directness	Limitations of study
Tekgul et al., 2006	Cohort study, retrospective analysis N=89	Neurological examination and neurodevelopmental testing after discharge and at 12 to 18 months	Prognostic value of seizure etiology, neurological examination, EEG and neuroimaging	good	good	useful	Retrospective, no control group. Outcome was limited to the early psychomotor development (18 months)
Ronen et al., 2007	Population-based study, prospective cohort study, clinical follow-up N=82/90	Prognostic value of seizure type, gestational age at delivery, birth weight, NS etiology, neonatal EEG and number of AED	Long term outcome: favourable with normal neurological and cognitive status, poor, (physical disability, cognitive impairment, learning disability, post-neonatal epilepsy)	good	Inconsistency in terms of brain maturity (both preterm and full term newborns included) and in term of type of seizures	very useful	Imaging findings not considered as separate prognostic factor. Included infants with generalized myoclonic events without EEG confirmation
Pisani et al., 2007	Cohort, prospective study N=106	Evaluation of status epilepticus and recurrent NS for neurological outcome, assessed at 24 months of corrected age. Impact of clinical factors (gestational age, birth weight, cerebral ultrasound findings). General development was assessed using Griffith's Mental development Scale	General development: normal or abnormal; neurodevelopmental outcome was classified as favourable or adverse (death, cerebral palsy, developmental delay, epilepsy, blindness or deafness)	moderate	Inconsistency in terms of brain maturity (both preterm and full term newborns included) and in term of type of seizures	Doesn't really answer question, but implied control of status and repeated neonatal seizures could reflect better outcome	All studied subjects had symptomatic NS, which usually reflects severe acute or chronic neurological injury; the high percentage of unfavourable outcome may be result of severe CNS involvement
Iype et al., 2008	Prospective cohort study, clinical follow-up over 2-8 months	Prognostic value of NS etiology, EEG (normal *vs.* interictal discharges), gestational age at delivery, birth weight	Favourable or poor in terms of mortality, neurological status and post-neonatal epilepsy	moderate	Inconsistency in terms of brain maturity type of seizures, and EEG confirmation	Useful for the prediction of early psychomotor development in newborn from the setting in a developing country	Seizures were recognized rather clinically than by EEG, short follow-up (2-8 months) is insufficient for diagnosis of mild motor and cognitive deficits and later onset of epilepsy
Pisani et al., 2008a	Prospective cohort study, clinical follow-up over 2-8 months N=51	Risk factors, etiology and type of NS, EEG activity, cerebral US scans	Favourable or poor in terms of mortality, neurological impairment and post-neonatal epilepsy	moderate	moderate	Useful for early psychomotor development in preterm babies of different degree of brain immaturity	It is difficult to distinguish the effects of NS on immature brain from influence of immaturity per se. The long term prognostic component was missing

References

Aggarwal P et al. (1998). Clinical predictors of outcome in hypoxic ischaemic encephalopathy in term neonates. *Annals of Tropical Paediatrics*, 18:117-121.

Ajayi OA, Oyaniyi OT, Chike-Obi UD (1998). Adverse effects of early phenobarbital administration in term newborns with perinatal asphyxia. *Tropical Medicine & International Health*, 3:592-595.

Alcover-Bloch E, Campistol J, Iriondo-Sanz M (2004). Neonatal seizures, our experience. *Revue Neurologique*, 38:808-812.

Andre M, Matisse N, Vert P, Debruille C (1988). Neonatal seizures - recent aspects. *Neuropediatrics*, 19:201-7.

Armstrong DL, Battin MR (2001). Pervasive seizures caused by hypoxic-ischemic encephalopathy: treatment with intravenous paraldehyde. *Journal of Child Neurology*, 16:915-7.

Atkins D et al. (2004). Systems for grading the quality of evidence and the strength of recommendations I: critical appraisal of existing approaches. *The GRADE Working Group. BMC Health Services Research*, 4:38.

Bartha AI et al. (2007). Neonatal seizures: multicenter variability in current treatment practices. *Pediatric Neurology*, 37:85-90.

Been JV et al. (2005). Epidemiology of pyridoxine dependent seizures in the Netherlands. *Archives of Diseases in Childhood*, 90:1293-6.

Bergman I et al. (1983). Outcome in neonates with convulsions treated in an intensive care unit. *Annals of Neurology*, 14:642-7.

Boylan GB et al. (1999). Outcome of electroclinical, electrographic, and clinical seizures in the newborn infant. *Developmental Medicine and Child Neurology*, 41:819-25.

Boylan GB et al. (2002). Phenobarbitone, neonatal seizures, and video-EEG. *Archives of Disease in Childhood-Fetal and Neonatal Edition*, 86:F165-70.

Boylan GB et al. (2004). Second-line anticonvulsant treatment of neonatal seizures: a video-EEG monitoring study. *Neurology*, 62:486-488.

Brod SA et al. (1988). Predictors of success for drug discontinuation following neonatal seizures. *Pediatric Neurology*, 4:13-7.

Brown JK, Cockburn F, Forfar JO (1972). Clinical and chemical correlates in convulsions of the newborn. *Lancet*, 1:135-9.

Brunquell PJ et al. (2002). Prediction of outcome based on clinical seizure type in newborn infants. *Journal of Pediatrics*, 140:707-12.

Burke JB (1954). The prognostic significance of neonatal convulsions. *Archives of Disease in Childhood*, 29:342-5.

Bye AM, Flanagan D (1995). Spatial and temporal characteristics of neonatal seizures. *Epilepsia*, 36:1009-16.

Bye AM et al. (1997). Outcome of neonates with electrographically identified seizures, or at risk of seizures. *Pediatric Neurology*, 16:225-31.

Caraballo RH et al. (2004). Symptomatic occipital lobe epilepsy following neonatal hypoglycemia. *Pediatric Neurology*, 31:24-9.

Carrascosa MC et al. (1996). Neonatal convulsions in health care. I. Incidence, etiology and clinical aspects. *Revue Neurologique*, 24:1258-62.

Castro Conde JR et al. (2005). Midazolam in neonatal seizures with no response to phenobarbital. *Neurology*, 64:876-879.

Clancy RR, Legido A (1991). Postnatal epilepsy after EEG-confirmed neonatal seizures. *Epilepsia*, 32:69-76.

Co JP et al. (2007). Proposal of an algorithm for diagnosis and treatment of neonatal seizures in developing countries. *Epilepsia*, 48:1158-1164.

Combes JC et al. (1975). Neonatal convulsions. Sudden onset and prognostic criteria. Apropos of 129 observation. *Pédiatrie*, 30:477-92.

Connell J et al. (1989). Clinical and EEG response to anticonvulsants in neonatal seizures. *Archives of Disease in Childhood*, 64:459-64.

Craig WS (1960). Convulsive movements occurring in the first 10 days of life. *Archives of Disease in Childhood*, 35:336-44.

Curtis PD et al. (1988). Neonatal seizures: the Dublin Collaborative Study. *Archives of Disease in Childhood*, 63:1065-8.

Dennis J (1978). Neonatal convulsions: aetiology, late neonatal status and long-term outcome. *Developmental Medicine and Child Neurology*, 20:143-8.

Derham RJ, Matthews TG, Clarke TA (1985). Early seizures indicate quality of perinatal care. *Archives of Disease in Childhood*, 60:809-13.

Domenech-Martinez E et al. (2003). Neonatal convulsions: influence of the electroencephalographic pattern and the response to treatment on the outcome. *Revue Neurologique*, 37:413-420.

Dreyfus-Brisac C et al. (1981). Convulsions in neonates. Clinical, electrographic, etiopathogenic and prognostic aspects. *Revue d'électroencéphalographie et de neurophysiologie clinique*, 11:367-78.

Ellison PH, Largent JA, Bahr JP (1981). A scoring system to predict outcome following neonatal seizures. *Journal of Pediatrics*, 99:455-9.

Eriksson M, Zetterström R (1979). Neonatal convulsions. Incidence and causes in the Stockholm area. *Acta Paediatrica Scandinavica*, 68:807-11.

Fischer K, Baarsma R (1996). Treatment of convulsions in newborn infants. *Nederlands tijdschrift voor geneeskunde*, 140:1557-60.

Foley ME et al. (2005). Term neonatal asphyxial seizures and peripartum deaths: lack of correlation with a rising cesarean delivery rate. *American Journal of Obstetrics and Gynecology*, 192:102-8.

Gal P, Boer HR (1982). Early discontinuation of anticonvulsants after neonatal seizures: a preliminary report. *Southern Medical Journal*, 75:298-300.

Garcias Da Silva LF, Nunes ML, Da Costa JC (2004). Risk factors for developing epilepsy after neonatal seizures. *Pediatric Neurology*, 30:271-7.

Gherpelli JL et al. (1992). Discontinuing medication in epileptic children: a study of risk factors related to recurrence. *Epilepsia*, 33:681-6.

Gilstrap LC 3rd et al. (1989). Diagnosis of birth asphyxia on the basis of fetal pH, Apgar score, and newborn cerebral dysfunction. *American Journal of Obstetrics and Gynecology*, 161:825-30.

Goldaber KG et al. (1991). Pathologic fetal acidemia. *Obstetrics and Gynecology*, 78:1103-7.

Goldberg HJ (1983). Neonatal convulsions - A 10-year review. *Archives of Disease in Childhood*, 58:976-8.

Graham EM, Holcroft CJ, Blakemore KJ (2002). Evidence of intrapartum hypoxia-ischemia is not present in the majority of cases of neonatal seizures. *Journal of Maternal-Fetal & Neonatal Medicine*, 12:123-6.

Guillet R, Kwon J (2007). Seizure Recurrence and Developmental Disabilities After Neonatal Seizures: Outcome Are Unrelated to Use of Phenobarbital Prophylaxis. *Journal of Child Neurology*, 22:389-395.

Gunn AJ, Gunn TR (1997). Changes in risk factors for hypoxic-ischaemic seizures in term infants. *The Australian & New Zealand journal of obstetrics & gynecology*, 37:36-9.

Gunn T, Cable G (1984). Neonatal seizures: aetiology and outcome. *The New Zealand Medical Journal*, 97:898-900.

Hall DA et al. (2006). Maternal risk factors for term neonatal seizures: population-based study in Colorado, 1989-2003. *Journal of Child Neurology*, 21:795-8.

Hall RT, Hall FK, Daily DK (1998). High-dose phenobarbital therapy in term newborn infants with severe perinatal asphyxia: a randomized, prospective study with three-year follow-up. *Journal of Pediatrics*, 132:345-348.

Hellstrom-Westas L et al. (1988). Lidocaine for treatment of severe seizures in newborn infants. I. Clinical effects and cerebral electrical activity monitoring. *Acta Paediatrica Scandinavica*, 77:79-84.

Holden KR, Mellits ED, Freeman JM (1982). Neonatal seizures. I. Correlation of prenatal and perinatal events with outcomes. *Pediatrics*, 70:165-76.

Hon EK, Bourchier D (1991). Overt neonatal seizures: outcome at one year. *The New Zealand Medical Journal*, 104:400-401.

Hosain S et al. (2003). Apneic seizures in infants: role of continuous EEG monitoring. *Clinical Electroencephalography*, 34:197-200.

Hu KC et al. (2003). Continuous midazolam infusion in the treatment of uncontrollable neonatal seizures. *Acta Paediatrica Taiwanica*, 44:279-81.

Idro R et al. (2008). The incidence, aetiology and outcome of acute seizures in children admitted to a rural Kenyan district hospital. *BMC Pediatrics*, 8:8-5.

Iype M et al. (2008). The newborn with seizures – A follow-up study. *Indian Pediatrics*, 45:749-752.

Jawadekar YM et al. (1992). A study of phenobarbital and dilantin in neonatal seizures. *Indian Journal of Pediatrics*, 59:729-34.

Keen JH, Lee D (1973). Sequelae of neonatal convulsions. Study of 112 infants. *Archives of Disease in Childhood*, 48:542-6.

Keeney SE, Adcock EW, McArdle CB (1991). Prospective observations of 100 high-risk neonates by high-field (1.5 Tesla) magnetic resonance imaging of the central nervous system. II. Lesions associated with hypoxic-ischemic encephalopathy. *Pediatrics*, 87:431-8.

Kerr SL et al. (1990). Sequential use of standard and ambulatory EEG in neonatal seizures. *Pediatric Neurology*, 6:159-62.

Khan RL et al. (2008). Predictive value of sequential electroencephalogram (EEG) in neonates with seizures and its relation to neurological outcome. *Journal of Child Neurology*, 23:144-50.

Kohelet D et al. (2004). Israel Neonatal Network. Risk factors for neonatal seizures in very low birthweight infants: population-based survey. *Journal of Child Neurology*, 19:123-8.

Krishnamoorthy KS et al. (2000). Diffusion-weighted imaging in neonatal cerebral infarction: clinical utility and follow-up. *Journal of Child Neurology*, 15:592-602.

Kumar A, Gupta A, Talukdar B (2007). Clinico-etiological and EEG profile of neonatal seizures. *Indian Journal of Pediatrics*, 74:33-7.

Labrecque D, Gal P, Sharpless MK (1984). Neonatal seizure recurrence following discontinuation of phenobarbital. *Clinical Pharmacy*, 3:649-52.

Langevin P (1974). Convulsions in the neonatal period. Evaluation of 21 cases. *Union Medical du Canada*, 103:465-9.

Lanska MJ, Lanska DJ, Baumann RJ (1994). False-positive reports of neonatal seizures on birth certificates. *American Journal of Public Health*, 84:1522.

Lanska MJ et al. (1995). A population-based study of neonatal seizures in Fayette County, Kentucky. *Neurology*, 45:724-32.

Lanska MJ, Lanska DJ (1996). Neonatal seizures in the United States: results of the National Hospital Discharge Survey, 1980-1991. *Neuroepidemiology*, 15:117-25.

Lanska MJ et al. (1996). Interobserver variability in the classification of neonatal seizures based on medical record data. *Pediatric Neurology*, 15:120-3.

Laroia N et al. (1998). EEG background as predictor of electrographic seizures in high-risk neonates. *Epilepsia*, 39:545-51.

Legido A, Clancy RR, Berman PH (1991). Neurologic outcome after electroencephalographically proven neonatal seizures. *Pediatrics*, 88:583-96.

Leveno KJ, Cunningham FG, Pritchard JA (1989). Cesarean section: the House of Horne revisited. *American Journal of Obstetrics and Gynecoly*, 160:78-9.

Lien JM et al. (1995). Term early-onset neonatal seizures: obstetric characteristics, etiologic classifications, and perinatal care. *Obstetrics and Gynecology*, 85:163-9.

Malik BA et al. (2005). Seizures etiology in the newborn period. *Journal of the College of Physicians and Surgeons Pakistan*, 15:786-90.

Maynard R, Garrel S (1983). Seizures in the newborn infant; value of polygraphy. *Revue d'Electroencéphalographie et de Neurophysiologie Clinique*, 13:219-23.

Maytal J, Novak GP, King KC (1991). Lorazepam in the treatment of refractory neonatal seizures. *Journal of Child Neurology*, 6:319-23.

McBride MC, Laroia N, Guillet R (2000). Electrographic seizures in neonates correlate with poor neurodevelopmental outcome. *Neurology*, 55:506-513.

Mclnerny TK, Schubert WK (1969). Prognosis of neonatal seizures. *American Journal of Diseases of Children*, 117:261-4.

Mclntire DD et al. (1999). Birth weight in relation to morbidity and mortality among newborn infants. *New England Journal of Medicine*, 340:1234-8.

Mellits ED, Holden KR, Freeman JM (1982). Neonatal seizures. II. A multivariate analysis of factors associated with outcome. *Pediatrics*, 70:177-85.

Ment LR, Freedman RM, Ehrenkranz RA (1982). Neonates with seizures attributable to perinatal complications: computed tomographic evaluation. *American Journal of Diseases of Children*, 136:548-50.

Mercuri E et al. (1995). Ischaemic and haemorrhagic brain lesions in newborns with seizures and normal Apgar scores. *Archives of Disease in Childhood - Fetal and Neonatal Edition*, 73:F67-74.

Miller SP et al. (2002). Seizure-associated brain injury in term newborns with perinatal asphyxia. *Neurology*, 58:542-548.

Minchom P et al. (1987). Antecedents and outcome of very early neonatal seizures in infants born at or after term. *British Journal of Obstetrics and Gynaecology*, 94:431-9.

Mizrahi EM, Kellaway P (1987). Characterization and classification of neonatal seizures. *Neurology*, 37:1837-44.

Murray DM et al. (2008). Defining the gap between electrographic seizure burden, clinical expression and staff recognition of neonatal seizures. *Archives of Disease in Childhood - Fetal and Neonatal Edition*, 93:F187-91.

Nunes ML et al. (2008). Neurological outcome of newborns with neonatal seizures: a cohort study in a tertiary university hospital. *Arquivos de Neuro-Psiquiatria*, 66:168-74.

Okan N et al. (1995). The prevalence of neurological disorders among children in Gemlik (Turkey). *Developmental Medicine and Child Neurology*, 37:597-603.

Ortibus EL, Sum JM, Hahn JS (1996). Predictive value of EEG for outcome and epilepsy following neonatal seizures. *Electroencephalography and Clinical Neurophysiology*, 98:175-85.

Painter MJ et al. (1999). Phenobarbital compared with phenytoin for the treatment of neonatal seizures. *New England Journal of Medicine*, 341:485-489.

Patterson CA et al. (1989). Antenatal and intrapartum factors associated with the occurrence of seizures in term infant. *Obstetrics and Gynecology*, 74:361-5.

Perlman JM, Risser R (1996). Can asphyxiated infants at risk for neonatal seizures be rapidly identified by current high-risk markers?. *Pediatrics*, 97:456-62.

Pezzani C et al. (1986). Neonatal electroencephalography during the first twenty-four hours of life in full-term newborn infants. *Neuropediatrics*, 17:11-8.

Pisani F et al. (2007). Neonatal status epilepticus *vs.* recurrent neonatal seizures: clinical findings and outcome. *Neurology*, 69:2177-85.

Pisani F et al. (2008a). Preterm infants with video-EEG confirmed seizures: outcome at 30 months of age. *Brain & Development*, 30:20-30.

Pisani F et al. (2008b). Neonatal seizures: relation of ictal video-electroencephalography (EEG) findings with neurodevelopmental outcome. *Journal of Child Neurology*, 23:394-8.

Plouin P et al. (1981). Neonatal status epilepticus of unknown etiology. *Revue d'Electroencéphalographie et de Neurophysiologie Clinique*, 11:385-9.

Radvanyi-Bouvet MF et al. (1985). Seizures and electrical discharges in premature infants. *Neuropediatrics*, 16:143-8.

Rennie JM, Boylan GB (2003). Neonatal seizures and their treatment. *Current Opinion in Neurology*, 16:177-81.

Rey E et al. (1990). Intravenous lidocaine in the treatment of convulsions in the neonatal period: monitoring plasma levels. *Therapeutic Drug Monitoring*, 12:316-20.

Rollins NK et al. (1994). The role of early MR in the evaluation of the term infant with seizures. *American Journal of Neuroradiology*, 15:239-48.

Ronen GM, Penney S, Andrews W (1999). The epidemiology of clinical neonatal seizures in Newfoundland: a population-based study. *Journal of Pediatrics*, 134:71-5.

Ronen GM et al. (2007). Long-term prognosis in children with neonatal seizures: a population-based study. *Neurology*, 69:1816-22.

Rose AL, Lombroso CT (1970). A study of clinical, pathological, and electroencephalographic features in 137 full-term babies with a long-term follow-up. *Pediatrics*, 45:404-25.

Rossiter EJ et al. (1977). Convulsions in the first three years of life. *Medical Journal of Australia*, 2:735-40.

Rowe JC et al. (1985). Prognostic value of the electroencephalogram in term and preterm infants following neonatal seizures. *Electroencephalography and Clinical Neurophysiology*, 60:183-96.

Rufo-Campos M et al. (2000). Cerebral seizures in neonatal period: semiology, evolution and factors of influence. *Revue Neurologique*, 31:301-6.

Saliba RM et al. (1999). Incidence of neonatal seizures in Harris County, Texas, 1992-1994. *American Journal of Epidemiololgy*, 150:763-9.

Saliba RM et al. (2001). Risk factors for neonatal seizures: a population-based study, Harris County, Texas, 1992-1994. *American Journal of Epidemiololgy*, 154:14-20.

Sankar MJ et al. (2007). Seizures in the newborn. *All India Institute of Medical Sciences (AIIMS) – Neuroscience Intensive Care Unit (NICO) protocols.*

Scarpa P et al. (1983). Criteria for discontinuing neonatal seizure therapy: a long-term appraisal. *Brain & Developement*, 5:541-8.

Scher MS et al. (1993). Electrographic seizures in preterm and full-term neonates: clinical correlates, associated brain lesions, and risk for neurologic sequelae. *Pediatrics*, 91:128-34.

Schulte FJ (1966). Neonatal convulsions and their relation to epilepsy in early childhood. *Developmental Medicine and Child Neurology*, 8:381-92.

Seay AR, Bray PF (1977). Significance of seizures in infants weighing less than 2,500 grams. *Archives of Neurology*, 34:381-2.

Shany E, Benzaqen O, Watemberg N (2007). Comparison of continuous drip of midazolam or lidocaine in the treatment of intractable neonatal seizures. *Journal of Child Neurology*, 22:255-9.

Sheth RD et al. (1996). Midazolam in the treatment of refractory neonatal seizures. *Clinical Neuropharmacology*, 19:165-70.

Sheth RD (1998). Frequency of neurologic disorders in the neonatal intensive care unit. *Journal of Child Neurology*, 13:424-8.

Sheth RD, Hobbs GR, Mullett M (1999). Neonatal seizures: incidence, onset, and aetiology by gestational age. *Journal of Perinatology*, 19:40-3.

Singh D, Kumar P, Narang A (2005). A randomized controlled trial of phenobarbital in neonates with hypoxic-ischemic encephalopathy. *Journal of Maternal-Fetal & Neonatal Medicine*, 18:391-395.

Staudt F (1990). The prognosis of convulsions in the newborn - the place of EEG in comparison with Echoencephalography. *EEG-EMG Zeitschrift für Elektroenzephalographie, Elektromyographie und verwandte Gebiete*, 21:118-25.

Strober JB, Bienkowski RS, Maytal J (1997). The incidence of acute and remote seizures in children with intraventricular hemorrhage. *Clinical Pediatrics*, 36:643-7.

Tekgul H et al. (2006). The current etiologic profile and neurodevelopmental outcome of seizures in term newborn infants. *Pediatrics*, 117:1270-80.

Temple CM et al. (1995). Neonatal seizures: long-term outcome and cognitive development among 'normal' survivors. *Developmental Medicine and Child Neurology*, 37:109-18.

Tharp BR, Cukier F, Monod N (1981). The prognostic value of the electroencephalogram in premature infants. *Electroencephalography and Clinical Neurophysiology*, 51:219-36.

Toet MC et al. (2005). Postneonatal epilepsy following amplitude-integrated EEG-detected neonatal seizures. *Pediatric Neurology*, 32:241-7.

Tsuboi T (1988). Prevalence and incidence of epilepsy in Tokyo. *Epilepsia*, 29:103-10.

Tudehope DI et al. (1988). Clinical spectrum and outcome of neonatal convulsions. *Australian Paediatric Journal*, 24:249-53.

van Leuven K et al. (2004). Midazolam and amplitude-integrated EEG in asphyxiated full-term neonates. *Acta Paediatrica*, 93:1221-7.

van Rooij LG et al. (2007). Neurodevelopmental outcome in term infants with status epilepticus detected with amplitude-integrated electroencephalography. *Pediatrics*, 120:354-63.

van Zeben-van der Aa DM et al. (1990). Neonatal seizures in very preterm and very low birthweight infants: mortality and handicaps at two years of age in a nationwide cohort. *Neuropediatrics*, 21:62-5.

Vargas-Origel A et al. (2004). Prevention of hypoxic-ischemic encephalopathy with high-dose, early phenobarbital therapy. *Gaceta médica de México*, 140:147-153.

Watkins A et al. (1988). Significance of seizures in very low-birthweight infants. *Developmental Medicine and Child Neurology*, 30:162-9.

Zalneraitis EL (1987). Diagnosis, significance, and treatment of neonatal seizures. *Rhode Island Medical Journal*, 70:347-54.

Appendix:
Search strategy of the literature

Search strategy of the literature

Search methods for identification of studies

The following databases were searched:

a) Cochrane Central Register of Controlled Trials (CENTRAL, The Cochrane Library, Issue 3, 2008: http://www3.interscience.wiley.com/cgi-bin/mrwhome/106568753/HOME?CRETRY=1&SRETRY=0)
b) MEDLINE any date (http://www.ncbi.nlm.nih.gov/sites/entrez)
c) Cabi Global Health database (http://www.cabi.org/home.asp)
d) National Library of Medicine (NLM) Gateway (http://gateway.nlm.nih.gov/gw/Cmd)
e) Centre for Reviews and Dissemination (CRD); web site: http://www.crd.york.ac.uk/crdweb/ (DARE: Database of Abstracts of Reviews of Effects plus NHS)
f) International registers of ongoing clinical trials ISRCTN (http://www.controlled-trials.com/isrctn/)
g) Embase (http://www.embase.com/)
h) Ovid MEDLINE database (http://gateway.ovid.com/autologin.html). Studies from 1950 to end of week 3 Nov 2008
i) Abstracts of annual meetings of Society of Pediatric Academic Societies 2000-2008 (http://www.abstracts2view.com/pasall)
j) A bibliographic database of Indian biomedical journals (http://indmed.nic.in/)
k) Manual search of abstracts of annual meetings of National Neonatology Forum of India
l) Wiley Inter Science journals database was searched
m) National Guidelines Clearinghouse was searched matching some of the keywords
n) Hand search within the International journals and Congress/Conference proceedings, and reference lists of the retrieved papers/studies (http://www.who.int/hinari/en/)

Search terms

The electronic search strategy involved keywords, using the search fields of abstract, MeSH subject heading, exploded subject heading, subject heading word, text word and title. The following key words were used:

- seizures
- convulsions
- newborn
- neonate
- treatment
- anticonvulsant drugs
- neuro* examination
- clinic*examination
- hypocalcaemia
- meningitis
- herpes simplex
- outcomes
- EEG
- predicting factors
- phenytoin
- phenobarbital
- midazolam
- diazepam
- lidocaine/lignocaine
- term
- preterm
- hypoglycaemia
- septicaemia
- pyridoxine
- prognosis
- neurodevelopment
- long-term
- diagnostic tests

Moreover, combinations of the above terms were used, employing the search fields of abstract, MeSH subject heading, exploded subject heading, subject heading word, text word and title.

Limits

Human, English, Clinical Trial, Meta Analysis, Practice Guideline, Randomised Controlled Trial, Review, Comparative study, Consensus Development Conference, NIH, Controlled Clinical trial, English abstract and Multicenter study.
And combinations with these key words.
Limitations: Clinical trial
Due to the paucity of documents retrieved with the above mentioned limitations, the search was repeated several times excluding some of the limitations.

a) Cochrane Central Register of Controlled Trials

CENTRAL, The Cochrane Library, Issue 3, 2008 (http://www3.interscience.wiley.com/cgi-bin/mrwhome/106568753/HOME?CRETRY=1&SRETRY=0),
Cochrane Controlled Trials Registry Search
Date: Issue 3, 2008
newborn, seizures, treatment and anticonvulsants.
The search retrieved 52 titles: 10 Cochrane reviews, one other review and 41 clinical trials.

b) MEDLINE any date (http://www.ncbi.nlm.nih.gov/sites/entrez)

Search Number 1

Limits: Humans, Clinical Trial, Randomized Controlled Trial, Systematic review, Newborn: birth-1 month

Search	Most Recent Queries	Time	Result
#15	Search (#3) AND (#14) Limits: Humans, Clinical Trial, Randomized Controlled Trial, Newborn: birth-1 month	14:31:51	243
#14	Search convulsions Limits: Humans, Clinical Trial, Randomized Controlled Trial, Review, Newborn: birth-1 month	14:30:51	861
#13	Search ((#1) AND (#7)) AND (#6) Limits: Humans, Clinical Trial, Randomized Controlled Trial, Newborn: birth-1 month	14:28:51	12
#12	Search (#1) AND (#7) Limits: Humans, Clinical Trial, Randomized Controlled Trial, Newborn: birth-1 month	14:28:27	17
#11	Search (((#1) AND) AND (#2)) AND (#5) Limits: Humans, Clinical Trial, Randomized Controlled Trial, Newborn: birth-1 month	14:27:41	18
#10	Search (#1) AND (#4) Limits: Humans, Clinical Trial, Randomized Controlled Trial, Newborn: birth-1 month	14:26:56	58
#9	Search (#1) AND (#3) Limits: Humans, Clinical Trial, Randomized Controlled Trial, Newborn: birth-1 month	14:26:28	56
#8	Search (#1) AND (#2) Limits: Humans, Clinical Trial, Randomized Controlled Trial, Newborn: birth-1 month	14:24:04	114
#7	Search phenytoin Limits: Humans, Clinical Trial, Randomized Controlled Trial, Newborn: birth-1 month	14:19:57	22
#6	Search phenobarbital Limits: Humans, Clinical Trial, Randomized Controlled Trial, Newborn: birth-1 month	14:19:48	129
#5	Search barbiturates Limits: Humans, Clinical Trial, Randomized Controlled Trial, Newborn: birth-1 month	14:19:38	153
#4	Search antiepileptic drugs Limits: Humans, Clinical Trial, Randomized Controlled Trial, Newborn: birth-1 month	14:19:19	316
#3	Search anticonvulsants Limits: Humans, Clinical Trial, Randomized Controlled Trial, Newborn: birth-1 month	14:19:06	314

#2	Search treatment Limits: Humans, Clinical Trial, Randomized Controlled Trial, Newborn: birth-1 month	14:18:51	10427
#1	Search seizures Limits: Humans, Clinical Trial, Randomized Controlled Trial, Newborn: birth-1 month	14:18:28	147

Search Number 2 (Repeated search in MEDLINE)
Limits: Humans, Clinical Trial, Randomized Controlled Trial, Review, Newborn: birth-1 month

Search	Most Recent Queries	Time	Result
#18	Search (#3) AND (#14) Limits: Humans, Clinical Trial, Randomized Controlled Trial, Newborn: birth-1 month	03:15:51	243
#17	Search convulsions Limits: Humans, Clinical Trial, Randomized Controlled Trial, Review, Newborn: birth-1 month	03:14:51	861
#16	Search (#3) AND (#6) Limits: Humans, Clinical Trial, Randomized Controlled Trial, Review, Newborn: birth-1 month	03:09:51	50
#15	Search (#12) AND (#11) AND (#6) AND (#4) Limits: Humans, Clinical Trial, Randomized Controlled Trial, Review, Newborn: birth-1 month	03:04:57	3
#14	Search (#1) AND (#11) AND (#5) Limits: Humans, Clinical Trial, Randomized Controlled Trial, Review, Newborn: birth-1 month	03:02:41	7
#13	Search midazolam Limits: Humans, Clinical Trial, Randomized Controlled Trial, Review, Newborn: birth-1 month	03:02:07	70
#12	Search phenytoin Limits: Humans, Clinical Trial, Randomized Controlled Trial, Review, Newborn: birth-1 month	03:02:00	129
#11	Search phenobarbital Limits: Humans, Clinical Trial, Randomized Controlled Trial, Review, Newborn: birth-1 month	03:01:48	322
#10	Search (#1)) AND (#4) AND (#6) Limits: Humans, Clinical Trial, Randomized Controlled Trial, Review, Newborn: birth-1 month	02:55:10	39
#9	Search (#3) AND (#6) Limits: Humans, Clinical Trial, Randomized Controlled Trial, Review, Newborn: birth-1 month	02:53:54	50
#8	Search (#1) AND (#3) AND (#5) Limits: Humans, Clinical Trial, Randomized Controlled Trial, Review, Newborn: birth-1 month	02:52:46	7
#7	Search (#1) AND (#2) AND (#6) Limits: Humans, Clinical Trial, Randomized Controlled Trial, Review, Newborn: birth-1 month	02:53:23	19
#6	Search duration Limits: Humans, Clinical Trial, Randomized Controlled Trial, Review, Newborn: birth-1 month	02:49:55	2159
#5	Search discharge Limits: Humans, Clinical Trial, Randomized Controlled Trial, Review, Newborn: birth-1 month	02:49:35	1078
#4	Search treatment Limits: Humans, Clinical Trial, Randomized Controlled Trial, Review, Newborn: birth-1 month	02:49:29	33688

#3	Search antiepileptic drugs Limits: Humans, Clinical Trial, Randomized Controlled Trial, Review, Newborn: birth-1 month	02:49:20	919
#2	Search anticonvulsants Limits: Humans, Clinical Trial, Randomized Controlled Trial, Review, Newborn: birth-1 month	02:49:09	902
#1	Search seizures Limits: Humans, Clinical Trial, Randomized Controlled Trial, Review, Newborn: birth-1 month	02:48:59	792

Search Number 3 (in PubMed)
Limits: Humans, All Infant: birth-23 months

Search	Most Recent Queries	Time	Result
#14	Search (#2) AND (#3) AND (#13) AND (#6) Limits: Humans, All Infant: birth-23 months	11:12:14	22
#13	Search antiepileptic drugs Limits: Humans, All Infant: birth-23 months	11:11:43	6698
#12	Search (#2) AND (#3) AND (#7) AND (#6) Limits: Humans, All Infant: birth-23 months	11:05:28	14
#11	Search (#2) AND (#3) AND (#5) Limits: Humans, All Infant: birth-23 months	11:04:13	22
#10	Search treatment Limits: Humans, All Infant: birth-23 months	11:02:49	337306
#9	Search (phenytoin) AND (#2) AND (#3) AND (#4)) AND (#6) Limits: Humans, All Infant: birth-23 months	11:01:35	4
#8	Search phenytoin Limits: Humans, All Infant: birth-23 months	11:01:13	949
#7	Search phenobarbital Limits: Humans, All Infant: birth-23 months	11:01:04	1733
#6	Search discharge Limits: Humans, All Infant: birth-23 months	11:00:49	7849
#5	Search anticonvulsants AND discharge Limits: Humans, All Infant: birth-23 months	11:00:38	79
#4	Search anticonvulsants Limits: Humans, All Infant: birth-23 months	11:00:29	6550
#3	Search newborn Limits: Humans, All Infant: birth-23 months	11:00:19	400680
#2	Search seizures Limits: Humans, All Infant: birth-23 months	11:00:06	10597
#1	Search Limits: Humans, All Infant: birth-23 months	10:59:52	725448

Date 08/11/2008, 13/11/2008 and 28/11/2008: Initially, the search was limited to clinical trials. However, only few papers were retrieved, most of which had to be excluded on the basis of the title. Therefore, the search was repeated without limit and 346 titles were retrieved.

Search	Most Recent Queries	Time	Result
#6	Search pyridoxine neonate seizure	12:12:10	120
#5	Search neonate seizure meningitis clinical	12:11:18	91
#3	Search septicemia neonate seizure clinical	12:09:55	58
#2	Search hypocalcemia neonate seizure clinical	12:09:22	30
#1	Search hypoglycemia neonate seizure clinical	12:08:45	47

Search	Most Recent Queries	Time	Results
#1	Search neonate seizure herpes	05:25:01	60

c) Cabi Global Health database (http://www.cabi.org/home.asp)

1 Neonatal screening for glutaryl-CoA dehydrogenase deficiency.
Lindner, M., Kölker, S., Schulze, A., Christensen, E. Greenberg, C. R., Hoffmann, G. F. / Journal of Inherited Metabolic Disease, 2004, Vol. 27, No. 6, pp. 851-859, 18 ref.
[Added:20050209]

2 Adverse effects of early phenobarbital administration in term newborns with perinatal asphyxia.
Ajayi, O. A., Oyaniyi, O. T., Chike-Obi, U. D. / Tropical Medicine and International Health, 1998, Vol. 3, No. 7, pp. 592-595, 13 ref.
[Added:19981205]

3 Phenylketonuria: contemporary screening and diagnosis.
Mabry, C. C. / Annals of Clinical and Laboratory Science, 1990, Vol. 20, No. 6, pp. 392-397, 18 ref.
[Added:19920829]

d) Search in NLM Gateway 1 (http://gateway.nlm.nih.gov/gw/Cmd)

Search History **Clear History**

NLM Gateway Search 1

Number	Search	Items Found	Actions
#25	Search: newborn and convulsions and anticonvulsants and Diazepam	195	View Results Delete
#24	Search: newborn and convulsions and anticonvulsants and Lidocaine	48	View Results Delete
#23	Search: newborn and convulsions and anticonvulsants and phenorbarbitone	0	View Results Delete
#22	Search: newborn and convulsions and anticonvulsants and phenytoin	226	View Results Delete
#21	Search: (newborn and seizures and term and treatment and Diazepam) and Phenytoin	62	View Results Delete
#20	Search: (newborn and seizures and preterm and treatment) and Clinic* examination	14	View Results Delete
#19	Search: (newborn and seizures and preterm and treatment) and Neuro* examination	7	View Results Delete
#18	Search: (newborn and seizures and preterm and treatment and phenytoin) and Neuro* examination	0	View Results Delete
#17	Search: (newborn and seizures and preterm and treatment and phenytoin) and Clinic* examination	0	View Results Delete
#16	Search: (neonates and convulsions and term and treatment) and Diazepam	386	View Results Delete
#15	Search: (neonates and convulsions and term and treatment) and Lidocaine	120	View Results Delete
#14	Search: (neonates and convulsions and term and treatment) and Phenorbarbitone	0	View Results Delete
#13	Search: (neonates and convulsions and term and treatment) and Phenytoin	131	View Results Delete
#12	Search: (neonates and convulsions and preterm and treatment) and Diazepam	33	View Results Delete

#11	Search: (neonates and convulsions and preterm and treatment) and Lidocaine	7	View Results Delete
#10	Search: (neonates and convulsions and preterm and treatment) and Phenorbarbitone	0	View Results Delete
#9	Search: (neonates and convulsions and preterm and treatment) and Phenytoin	14	View Results Delete
#8	Search: (newborn and seizures and term and treatment) and Phenytoin	102	View Results Delete
#7	Search: (newborn and seizures and term and treatment) and Phenorbarbital	0	View Results Delete
#6	Search: (newborn and seizures and term and treatment) and Phenorbarbitone	0	View Results Delete
#5	Search: (newborn and seizures and term and treatment) and Lidocaine	101	View Results Delete
#4	Search: (newborn and seizures and term and treatment) and Diazepam	305	View Results Delete
#3	Search: (newborn and seizures and preterm and treatment) and Diazepam	24	View Results Delete
#2	Search: (newborn and seizures and preterm and treatment) and Lidocaine	5	View Results Delete
#1	Search: (newborn and seizures and preterm and treatment) and phenorbarbital	0	View Results Delete

NLM Gateway search 2

Clinical trials 18 titles retrieved

Number	Search	Items Found	Actions
#8	Search: perinatal and seizures and anticonvulsants and discharge	18	View Results Delete
#7	Search: neonatal and seizures and anticonvulsants and discharge	66	View Results Delete
#6	Search: newborn and seizures and anticonvulsants and discharge	55	View Results Delete
#5	Search: newborn and seizures and phenytoin	275	View Results Delete
#4	Search: newborn and seizures and phenobarbital	682	View Results Delete
#3	Search: seizures and newborn and antiepileptic drugs	1100	View Results Delete
#2	Search: seizures and newborn and therapy	2968	View Results Delete
#1	Search: seizures and newborn and anticonvulsants	1070	View Results Delete

04. 11. 2008

Search in NLM Gateway (http://gateway.nlm.nih.gov/gw/Cmd)

Neonatal seizures and prognosis Summary: **1148** records found

Neonatal seizures and prognosis, clinical trials, reviews Summary: **57** records found

06.11.2008

Neonatal seizures and prognostic factors Summary: **69** records found

Neonatal seizures and prognostic factors, clinical trials Summary: **9** records found

Neonatal seizures and prognostic tests Summary: **27** records found

Neonatal seizures and prognostic tests, clinical trials Summary: **10** records found

105 Items. were selected

e) Centre for Reviews and Dissemination - CRD

(http://www.crd.york.ac.uk/crdweb/)

CRD (Centre for Review and Dissemination) consisting of DARE: Database of Abstracts of Reviews of Effects, *Structured abstracts of quality-assessed reviews* and National Institute for Health research (NHS)

Search history		Matching records
#1	neonatal seizures AND prognosis RESTRICT YR 1990 2008	0
#2	neonatal seizures AND prognosis AND factors AND tests RESTRICT YR 1970 2008	0

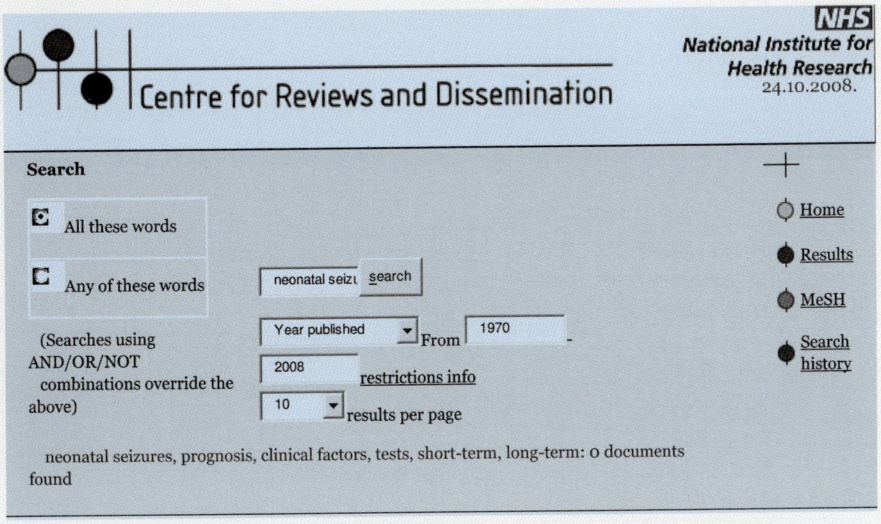

Search history		Matching records
#1	newborn AND seizures AND treatment RESTRICT YR 1998 2008	6

f) International registers of ongoing clinical trials ISRCTN

(http://www.controlled-trials.com/isrctn/)

Internet-based trials registers were searched for ongoing trials. The registers searched were: Trials Central (www.trialscentral.org) which is a database of clinical trials registers that gives access to Current Controlled Trials, made up of two registers, ISRCTN (a database of randomized controlled trials with an international randomized controlled trial number) and mRCT (metaRegister of controlled trials), a database combining registers of ongoing randomized controlled trials in all areas of healthcare. Trials Central also links to the Australasian Perinatal Trials Registry.

These registers were searched using keywords *neonate* and *seizure*.

International registers of ongoing clinical trials ISRCTN
http://www.controlled trials.com/isrctn/

30.09.2008 / 10.11.2008

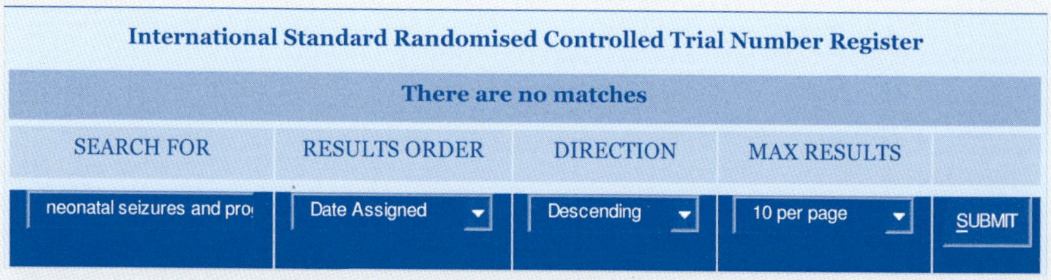

Internet-based trials registers (10.11.2008 and 30.09.2008) were searched twice for ongoing trials. These registers were searched using keywords *neonatal* and *seizures*; *neonatal seizures* and *prognosis*.

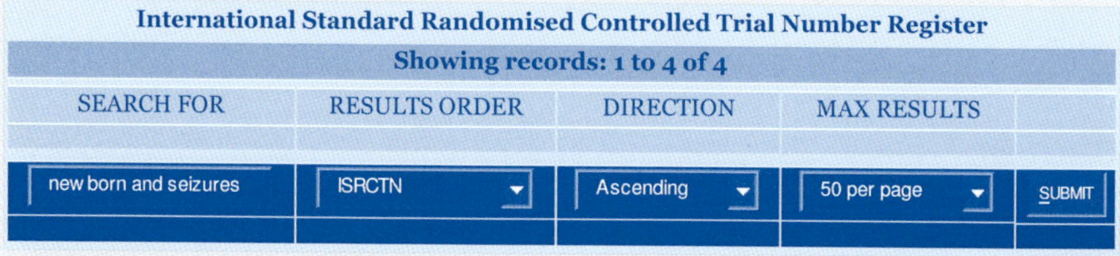

01	Effectiveness of sucrose analgesia in reducing pain responses in infants born to diabetic and non-diabetic mothers: A randomized controlled trial Date assigned: 15 August 2005
02	Levetiracetam (Keppra®) in neonates: safety of intravenous levetiracetam for neonates with seizures Date assigned: 11 April 2007
03	Minimizing needle poke pain in newborn infants with a pain relieving cream and sugar water Date assigned: 23 August 2007
04	Effect of timing of cord clamping on postnatal packed red blood cells value and clinical outcome in term newborns: a randomised controlled trial Date assigned: 02 March 2005

These registers were searched using keywords *neonatal* and *seizures*; *neonatal and seizure* and 7 trials retrieved:

01	Effectiveness of sucrose analgesia in reducing pain responses in infants born to diabetic and non-diabetic mothers: A randomized controlled trial Date assigned: 15 August 2005
02	Levetiracetam (Keppra®) in neonates: safety of intravenous levetiracetam for neonates with seizures Date assigned: 11 April 2007
03	Minimizing needle poke pain in newborn infants with a pain relieving cream and sugar water Date assigned: 23 August 2007
04	Effect of timing of cord clamping on postnatal packed red blood cells value and clinical outcome in term newborns: a randomised controlled trial Date assigned: 02 March 2005
05	Efficacy of zinc (given as an adjunct) in the treatment of severe and very severe pneumonia in hospitalised children 2 to 24 months of age Date assigned: 23 April 2007

06	The effect of treatment of neonatal electrographic seizures, detected with the continuous cerebral function monitoring, with respect to occurrence of post-neonatal epilepsy and neurodevelopmental outcome. Date assigned: 20 December 2005
07	Whole body hypothermia for the treatment of perinatal asphyxial encephalopathy Date assigned: 21 September 2000

Some of the titles were overlapped during the combined search.

g) Embase (http://www.embase.com/)

h) Ovid MEDLINE database (http://gateway.ovid.com/autologin.html).

Studies from 1950 to end of week 3 November 2008
Search History saved as "Neonatal seizures 1"

Search History (13 searches) (Click to expand) (Click to close)

	Searches	Results	Search Type	Display
#1	(neonate and seizures and phenobarbital).mp. [mp=title, original title, abstract, name of substance word, subject heading word]	24	Advanced	Display
#2	limit 1 to (abstracts and english language and humans)	22	Advanced	Display
#3	(neonate and seizures and phenytoin).mp. [mp=title, original title, abstract, name of substance word, subject heading word]	15	Advanced	Display
#4	(neonate and seizures and lidocaine).mp. [mp=title, original title, abstract, name of substance word, subject heading word]	4	Advanced	Display
#5	(neonate and seizures and diazepam).mp. [mp=title, original title, abstract, name of substance word, subject heading word]	6	Advanced	Display
#6	(newborn and phenobarbital and anticonvulsants).mp. [mp=title, original title, abstract, name of substance word, subject heading word]	257	Advanced	Display
#7	limit 6 to (abstracts and english language and humans)	160	Advanced	Display
#8	(newborn and phenytoin and anticonvulsants). mp. [mp=title, original title, abstract, name of substance word, subject heading word]	252	Advanced	Display
#9	limit 8 to (abstracts and english language and humans)	146	Advanced	Display
#10	(newborn and midazolam and anticonvulsants). mp. [mp=title, original title, abstract, name of substance word, subject heading word]	26	Advanced	Display
#11	(newborn and diazepam and anticonvulsants). mp. [mp=title, original title, abstract, name of substance word, subject heading word]	80	Advanced	Display
#12	limit 11 to (abstracts and english language and humans)	41	Advanced	Display
#13	(newborn and lidocaine and anticonvulsants). mp. [mp=title, original title, abstract, name of substance word, subject heading word]	22	Advanced	Display

Ovid *EEG*
Database: Ovid MEDLINE(R) 1950 to Present with Daily Update

Search Strategy:
1 seizures/ or seizures, febrile/ (35556)
2 seizure$1.ti,ab. (61915)
3 1 or 2 (77985)
4 exp Infant, Newborn/ (429018)
5 3 and 4 (5098)
6 (newborn or neonat$2).ti,ab. (207340)
7 3 and 6 (3452)
8 7 or 5 (6211)
9 exp Electroencephalography/ (108506)
10 (Electroencephalogra$3 or eeg$1).ti,ab. (53047)
11 10 or 9 (117394)
12 8 and 11 (1604)
13 limit 12 to yr="1980 - 2008" (1376)
14 from 13 keep 2 (1)
15 seizures/di or seizures, febrile/di (3153)
16 2 and di.fs. (14424)
17 16 or 15 (15441)
18 13 and 17 (733)
19 13 not 18 (643)
20 (outcome$1 or utility or value).ti,ab. (937651)
21 19 and 20 (157)
22 21 or 18 (890)
23 from 22 keep 1-500 (500)
24 from 22 keep 501-890 (390)

OVID ultrasound
Database: Ovid MEDLINE(R) 1950 to Present with Daily Update

Search Strategy:
1 seizures/ or seizures, febrile/ (35556)
2 seizure$1.ti,ab. (61915)
3 1 or 2 (77985)
4 exp Infant, Newborn/ (429018)
5 3 and 4 (5098)
6 (newborn or neonat$2).ti,ab. (207340)
7 3 and 6 (3452)
8 7 or 5 (6211)
9 exp Electroencephalography/ (108506)
10 (Electroencephalogra$3 or eeg$1).ti,ab. (53047)
11 10 or 9 (117394)
12 8 and 11 (1604)
13 limit 12 to yr="1980 - 2008" (1376)
14 from 13 keep 2 (1)
15 seizures/di or seizures, febrile/di (3153)
16 2 and di.fs. (14424)
17 16 or 15 (15441)
18 13 and 17 (733)
19 13 not 18 (643)
20 (outcome$1 or utility or value).ti,ab. (937651)
21 19 and 20 (157)
22 21 or 18 (890)
23 from 22 keep 1-500 (500)

24 from 22 keep 501-890 (390)
25 Magnetic Resonance Imaging/ (190329)
26 25 or mri.ti,ab. (210510)
27 26 and 17 (3891)
28 limit 27 to yr="1980 - 2008" (3891)
29 8 and 17 (1816)
30 26 and 29 (353)
31 from 30 keep 1-353 (353)
32 Tomography, X-Ray Computed/ (210791)
33 32 or ct.ti,ab. (267531)
34 33 and 29 (249)
35 from 34 keep 1-249 (249)
36 Ultrasonography/ or Ultrasonography, Doppler, Transcranial/ (63182)
37 ultrasound.ti,ab. (98222)
38 36 or 37 (140891)
39 38 and 29 (64)
40 limit 39 to yr="1980 - 2008" (64)
41 from 40 keep 1-64 (64)

OVID CT
Ovid Technologies, Inc. Email Service

Search for: 33 and 29
Results: 1-249
Database: Ovid MEDLINE(R) 1950 to Present with Daily Update

Search Strategy:
1 seizures/ or seizures, febrile/ (35556)
2 seizure$1.ti,ab. (61915)
3 1 or 2 (77985)
4 exp Infant, Newborn/ (429018)
5 3 and 4 (5098)
6 (newborn or neonat$2).ti,ab. (207340)
7 3 and 6 (3452)
8 7 or 5 (6211)
9 exp Electroencephalography/ (108506)
10 (Electroencephalogra$3 or eeg$1).ti,ab. (53047)
11 10 or 9 (117394)
12 8 and 11 (1604)
13 limit 12 to yr="1980 - 2008" (1376)
14 from 13 keep 2 (1)
15 seizures/di or seizures, febrile/di (3153)
16 2 and di.fs. (14424)
17 16 or 15 (15441)
18 13 and 17 (733)
19 13 not 18 (643)
20 (outcome$1 or utility or value).ti,ab. (937651)
21 19 and 20 (157)
22 21 or 18 (890)
23 from 22 keep 1-500 (500)
24 from 22 keep 501-890 (390)
25 Magnetic Resonance Imaging/ (190329)
26 25 or mri.ti,ab. (210510)
27 26 and 17 (3891)
28 limit 27 to yr="1980 - 2008" (3891)
29 8 and 17 (1816)

30 26 and 29 (353)
31 from 30 keep 1-353 (353)
32 Tomography, X-Ray Computed/ (210791)
33 32 or ct.ti,ab. (267531)
34 33 and 29 (249)
35 from 34 keep 1-249 (249)

OVID MRI

Database: Ovid MEDLINE(R) 1950 to Present with Daily Update

Search strategy:

1 seizures/ or seizures, febrile/ (35556)
2 seizure$1.ti,ab. (61915)
3 1 or 2 (77985)
4 exp Infant, Newborn/ (429018)
5 3 and 4 (5098)
6 (newborn or neonat$2).ti,ab. (207340)
7 3 and 6 (3452)
8 7 or 5 (6211)
9 exp Electroencephalography/ (108506)
10 (Electroencephalogra$3 or eeg$1).ti,ab. (53047)
11 10 or 9 (117394)
12 8 and 11 (1604)
13 limit 12 to yr="1980 - 2008" (1376)
14 from 13 keep 2 (1)
15 seizures/di or seizures, febrile/di (3153)
16 2 and di.fs. (14424)
17 16 or 15 (15441)
18 13 and 17 (733)
19 13 not 18 (643)
20 (outcome$1 or utility or value).ti,ab. (937651)
21 19 and 20 (157)
22 21 or 18 (890)
23 from 22 keep 1-500 (500)
24 from 22 keep 501-890 (390)
25 Magnetic Resonance Imaging/ (190329)
26 25 or mri.ti,ab. (210510)
27 26 and 17 (3891)
28 limit 27 to yr="1980 - 2008" (3891)
29 8 and 17 (1816)
30 26 and 29 (353)
31 from 30 keep 1-353 (353)

i) Abstracts of Annual meetings of Society of Pediatric Academic Societies 2000-2008 (http://www.abstracts2view.com/pasall)

j) A Bibliographic database of Indian biomedical journals (http://indmed.nic.in/)

k) Manual search of abstracts of annual meetings of National Neonatology Forum of India.

l) Wiley Inter Science database was searched.
There were 37 results for: "Prognosis of neonatal seizures in All Fields, in all subjects, in product type Journals"